28 Day

Simple Chair Yoga for Seniors and

Beginners *Over 60*

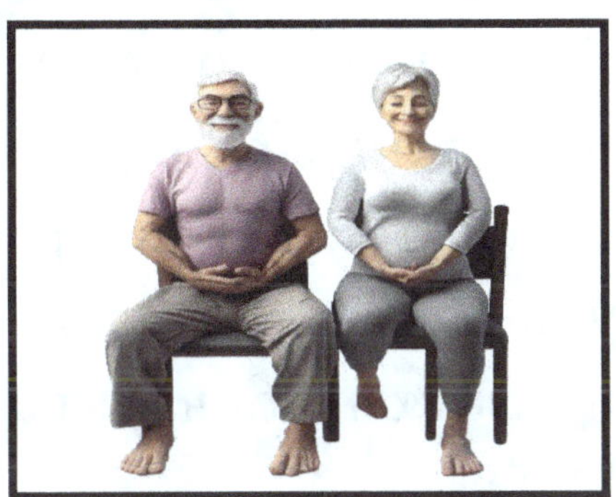

Improving Heart Health and Posture, Intermediate and Advanced Fitness Challenge for Quick Weight Loss through Essential Exercises

Valarie D. Flores

Copyright © 2024 Valarie D. Flores All rights reserved.

The copyright statement affirms the protected status of the book under copyright law, with Valarie D. Flores designated as the copyright owner. The inclusion of "All rights reserved" conveys that the book is not to be reproduced, distributed, or transmitted through any means without the explicit permission of the author, except in cases permitted under fair use exemptions as outlined by copyright law.

Table of Contents

28 Day workout planner

WEEKLY WORKOUT
PLANNER

DAY	STRENGHT TRAINING	CARDIO
MON		
TUE		
WED		
THU		
FR		
SAT		
SUN		

Notes:

WEEKLY WORKOUT
PLANNER

DAY	STRENGHT TRAINING	CARDIO
MON		
TUE		
WED		
THU		
FR		
SAT		
SUN		

Notes:

WEEKLY WORKOUT
PLANNER

DAY	STRENGHT TRAINING	CARDIO
MON		
TUE		
WED		
THU		
FR		
SAT		
SUN		

Notes:

WEEKLY WORKOUT
PLANNER

DAY	STRENGHT TRAINING	CARDIO
MON		
TUE		
WED		
THU		
FR		
SAT		
SUN		

Notes:

Introduction

Welcome

Welcome to "28 Days Simple Chair Yoga for Seniors and Beginners Over 60." This book is more than a guide;

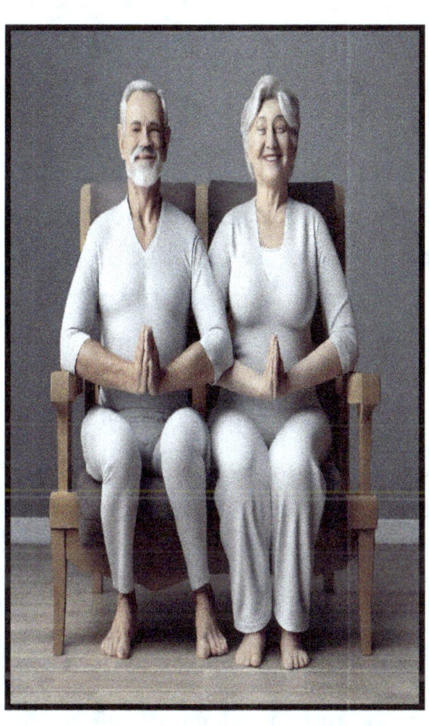

it's an invitation to embark on a deeply personal journey of rejuvenation and self-care. Imagine the story of Mary, a vibrant soul in her 60s, who, like many of us, found herself navigating the inevitable changes that come with aging. As she flipped through the pages of this very guide, filled with gentle poses and mindful breathing exercises, Mary found herself drawn to the possibility of reclaiming a sense of vitality and well-being that age seemed to have taken away.

Through tears of frustration and laughter of realization, Mary discovered the transformative power of chair yoga. She found solace in the simple joy of stretching her arms towards the sky, feeling a newfound strength in her core, and embracing the peace that comes from a deep, intentional breath. Each day, as she turned the pages and welcomed the gentle guidance within, Mary felt a sense of renewal seep into her being, awakening a vitality she thought had long since slipped away.

With each passing week, she noticed herself standing a little taller, feeling a little stronger, and approaching life with a renewed sense of grace and ease. The simple act of settling into her favorite chair became a sacred ritual of self-care, a testament to her unwavering commitment to her own well-being. This book is an embodiment of Mary's journey, offering a promise of hope, renewal, and the power of gentle movement for anyone who wishes to embrace the gifts of chair yoga.

So, as you turn the page and begin this 28-day journey, remember that you are not alone. You are part of a community of seekers and believers - like Mary - who have found solace, strength, and sanctuary in the simple practice of chair yoga. Here's to embracing the next chapter of your life with open arms, steady breath, and the gentle guidance of chair yoga.

Benefits of Chair Yoga for Seniors and Beginners

Chair yoga offers a myriad of benefits for seniors, making it a valuable and accessible wellness practice. These benefits encompass physical, mental, and emotional well-being, catering specifically to the unique needs and considerations of older individuals.

1. **Improved Flexibility and Mobility**: Chair yoga incorporates gentle stretching and movement, which can help seniors maintain or improve flexibility in their muscles and joints. This is especially beneficial for those with limited mobility or stiffness, as it encourages a wider range of motion.

2. **Enhanced Strength**: Despite being seated, chair yoga includes poses and exercises that engage various muscle groups, contributing to improved strength and stability. This is crucial for seniors in maintaining their independence and reducing the risk of falls.

3. **Better Posture and Balance**: Practicing chair yoga can help seniors develop better posture and balance, which are essential for daily activities and overall physical well-being. The focus on alignment and mindful

movement supports a more upright posture and reduces the risk of falls.

4. **Stress Reduction and Relaxation**: Through gentle breathing techniques and relaxation exercises, chair yoga offers seniors an opportunity to unwind and release tension. This can have a positive impact on mental well-being, promoting a sense of calm and reducing stress levels.

5. **Enhanced Mindfulness and Focus**: Chair yoga encourages participants to be present in the moment, fostering mindfulness and improved concentration. For seniors, this can be particularly valuable in maintaining mental acuity and cognitive function.

6. **Pain Management and Relief**: The gentle movements and stretches in chair yoga can contribute to reducing discomfort related to conditions such as arthritis, back pain, or stiffness. It offers a low-impact approach to managing and alleviating musculoskeletal issues.

7. **Social Connection**: Engaging in chair yoga classes or practices can provide seniors with a sense of community and social connection. This is important for combating feelings of isolation and fostering a supportive environment for overall well-being.

8. **Emotional Well-being:** Chair yoga promotes emotional health by providing an outlet for self-expression, self-care, and a sense of accomplishment. It can uplift spirits, reduce feelings of anxiety or depression, and enhance overall emotional resilience.

9. **Accessible Exercise**: Perhaps one of the most significant benefits of chair yoga for seniors is its accessibility. The use of a chair as a prop makes yoga achievable for individuals with limited mobility, balance concerns, or other physical limitations, ensuring that everyone can reap the rewards of a consistent yoga practice.

10. **Improved Sleep Quality**: By incorporating relaxation and gentle movements, chair yoga can contribute to improved sleep quality for seniors. Better sleep has a ripple effect on overall health and vitality, promoting a greater sense of well-being.

Chair yoga offers a holistic approach to wellness for seniors, addressing physical, mental, and emotional facets of their well-being. Its gentle nature, adaptability, and focus on mindfulness make it an invaluable practice for those seeking to maintain and enhance their vitality as they age.

How to Use This Book

1. **Introduction**: Start by reading the introduction attentively. Understand the author's perspective, the structure of the book, and the intended outcomes of the chair yoga program.

2. **Assess Your Needs**: Before starting the program, assess your own physical capabilities and any specific areas of concern. This will help you tailor the practice to your needs.

3. **Daily Structure**: As the title implies, the book likely lays out a 28-day program. Plan to dedicate a specific time each day for your chair yoga practice.

4. **Follow Each Day**: The book probably outlines specific yoga poses, movements, and sequences for each day. Follow each day's recommended practice as outlined in the book.

5. **Mindful Practice**: Engage mindfully with the chair yoga sequences. Pay attention to your breath, body alignment, and any sensations that arise during the practice.

6. **Recording Progress**: Consider keeping a journal to track your progress. Note any improvements in flexibility, strength, or overall well-being as you progress through the 28-day program.

7. **Seek Support**: If possible, practice with a partner or seek support from friends or family members who can participate or encourage you in your chair yoga journey.

8. **Modify as Needed**: Acknowledge that everyone's body is different. Feel free to modify the poses and movements as necessary to suit your comfort and abilities.

9. **Repetition and Consistency**: Don't be discouraged if certain poses feel challenging at first. Consistent practice over the 28 days can lead to improved comfort and proficiency.

10. **Post-Program Reflection**: After completing the 28-day program, take time to reflect on your journey, noting any physical or mental changes you've experienced.

By actively engaging with the chair yoga program, tracking your progress, and seeking support as needed, you can derive significant benefits from the book "28 Days Simple Chair Yoga for Senior Beginners Over 60."

Always remember to prioritize safety and listen to your body throughout your practice.

Week 1: Foundational Poses and Breathing Techniques

Day 1: Setting the Foundation

Setting the foundation in chair yoga involves establishing a strong understanding of fundamental

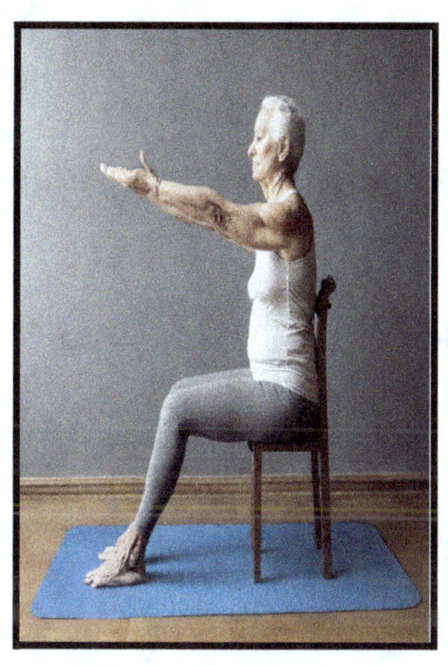

principles that will support your practice throughout the 28-day program. Here are some key points to consider when setting the foundation for your chair yoga practice:

1. **Breath Awareness**: Begin by cultivating an awareness of your breath. Understand the role of deep, diaphragmatic breathing in chair yoga, and how it can enhance relaxation and promote a sense of calm. Practice deep breathing exercises to connect with your breath and its ability to center and ground you.

2. **Proper Alignment**: Focus on aligning your body mindfully in each pose. Explore how to sit tall and engage your core while maintaining a sense of ease and comfort. Pay attention to the instructions for each pose, emphasizing the importance of alignment to prevent strain and promote stability.

3. **Modification and Adaptation**: Acknowledge that chair yoga is adaptable to individuals with varying levels of flexibility and mobility. Embrace the concept of modifying poses to suit your unique needs, using props or adjusting the intensity of the movements as necessary. This approach ensures that chair yoga can be accessible and beneficial for everyone.

4. **Mindful Movement**: Approach each movement with mindfulness. Be present in the sensations that arise as you transition between poses and explore the range of motion in your body. Cultivate a sense of mindfulness in your practice to deepen your mind-body connection.

5. **Respect Your Limitations**: Honor your body's limitations and avoid pushing yourself beyond a comfortable range of motion. Chair yoga is about gentle, safe movement, so practice in a way that feels supportive and nurturing for your body.

6. **Intentions and Mindset**: Consider setting an intention for your chair yoga practice. Whether it's to increase flexibility, reduce stress, or enhance overall well-being, having a clear intention can guide your focus and commitment throughout the program.

By establishing these foundational principles, you can build a solid framework for your chair yoga practice. Over time, these principles will become second nature, allowing you to experience the full benefits of the practice with confidence and ease. As you progress through the program, revisit these foundational elements regularly to deepen your understanding and refine your practice.

Day 2: Gentle Neck and Shoulder Stretches

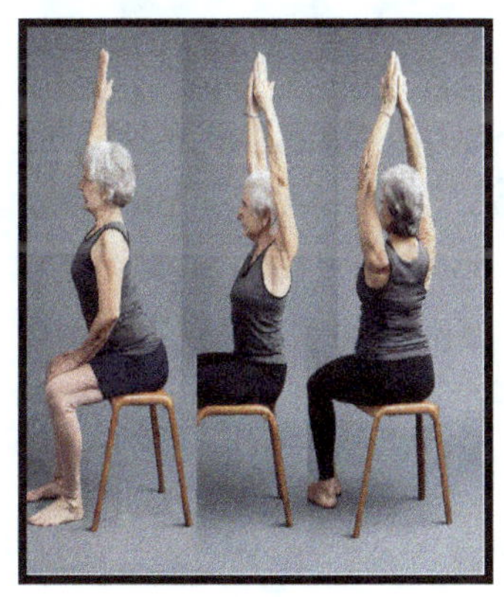

On the second day of your chair yoga journey, focusing on gentle neck and shoulder stretches can provide relief from tension and promote relaxation. Here are some suggested gentle neck and shoulder stretches:

1. **Neck Rolls**: While seated comfortably in your chair with your spine tall, slowly drop your chin towards your chest. From there, begin to roll your head to the right, bringing your right ear towards your right shoulder. Continue the circular motion by slowly rolling your head back and then to the left, bringing your left ear towards your left shoulder. Complete the circular motion by returning to the starting position. Perform this movement slowly and mindfully, allowing your neck muscles to relax and release any tightness.

2. **Shoulder Rolls**: Sit comfortably with your hands resting on your thighs. Inhale as you shrug your shoulders up towards your ears, feeling the gentle stretch in the shoulders and neck. Exhale as you roll your shoulders back and down, completing the circular motion. Repeat this several times, allowing your breath to guide the movement and release tension in the shoulders.

3. **Ear to Shoulder Stretch**: Sit up straight and tilt your head to the right, bringing your right ear towards your right shoulder. Use your right hand to gently apply a bit of extra pressure to deepen the stretch on the left side of your neck, being careful not to strain. Hold this stretch for a few deep breaths, then switch to the left side and repeat.

4. **Eagle Arms Stretch**: Extend your arms straight in front of you at shoulder height. Cross your right arm over the left, bringing the palms to touch if possible. If this is too intense, you can simply bring the backs of your hands together. Lift your elbows, feeling a stretch across the upper back and shoulders. Hold for a few breaths, then release and switch the crossing of your arms.

5. **Seated Neck Stretch**: Sit on the edge of your chair and hold onto the side of the seat with your right hand. Gently tilt your head to the left, bringing your left ear towards your left shoulder while keeping your right shoulder grounded. Feel a stretch along the right side of your neck. Hold for a few breaths, then switch to the other side.

As you move through these gentle stretches, remember to maintain a sense of ease and relaxation, allowing the tensions in your neck and shoulders to melt away. Focus on your breath and stay present with the sensations in your body. These stretches can be repeated as needed throughout the week to help alleviate stress and promote mobility in the neck and shoulders. Always listen to your body and modify the stretches as necessary to suit your comfort level.

Day 3: Seated Forward Bend

On the third seated forward bends are wonderful for stretching the lower back, hamstrings, and relieving tension in the spine. Here's how you can perform a seated forward bend:

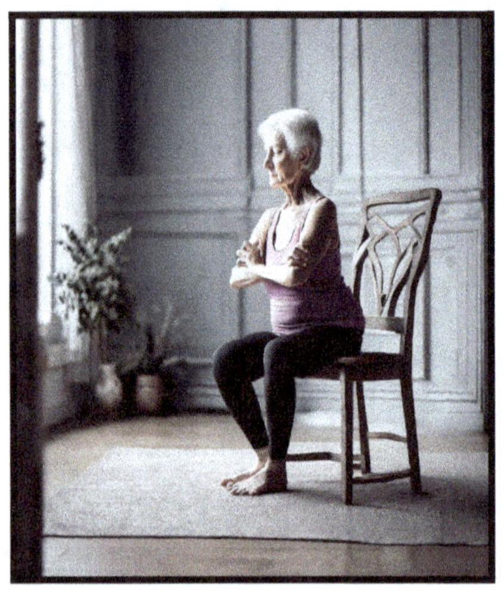

1. **Sit Up Straight**: Begin by sitting towards the front of your chair with your feet flat on the floor and hip-width apart. Sit up tall with your spine lengthened and your shoulders relaxed. Take a moment to center yourself and connect with your breath.

2. **Inhale and Lengthen**: As you inhale, extend your arms out to the sides and then up overhead. Reach towards the ceiling to elongate your spine and create space between each vertebra. Feel the gentle stretch along your sides as you reach upward.

3. **Exhale and Fold Forward**: As you exhale, slowly hinge at your hips and begin to fold forward from your

lower back, keeping your chest open. Lead with your chest and allow your hands to reach towards your feet or the floor in front of you. If you're unable to reach your feet, simply reach forward to where you feel a comfortable stretch. It's important not to force the stretch.

4. **Lengthen the Spine**: Once you have reached your maximum comfortable stretch, instead of focusing on touching your toes, focus on lengthening your spine. Imagine your belly button moving towards your thighs, and your chest moving toward your knees, which helps to elongate your spine and deepens the stretch.

5. **Relax and Breathe**: Once you have found your maximum stretch and lengthened your spine, relax your head, neck, and shoulders. Take slow, deep breaths as you hold the position, allowing your body to release any tension.

6. **Hold and Release**: Hold the position for several breaths, feeling the gentle stretch along your lower back and the backs of your legs. When you are ready to release the stretch, slowly inhale as you rise back up to a seated position, keeping your movements slow and deliberate.

Remember, the key to a seated forward bend is to focus on the lengthening of the spine and the breath, rather than straining to touch your toes. This approach will help you avoid unnecessary tension and allow for a more mindful and effective stretch. If you experience any discomfort or pain, ease out of the stretch and adjust your position as needed. This gentle and mindful approach to seated forward bends can be incorporated into your routine as needed to provide relief and relaxation for your lower back and hamstrings.

Day 4: Deep Breathing Exercises

On day 4 of deep breathing exercises, it's fantastic that you are incorporating this practice into your routine!

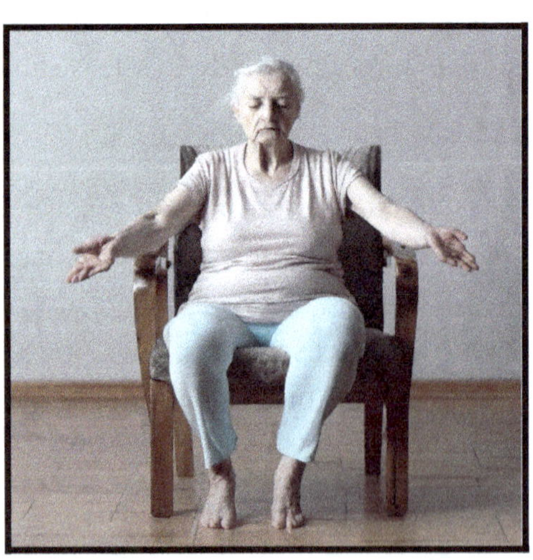

Deep breathing exercises can bring about a sense of calm and relaxation, while also benefiting your physical and emotional well-being. Here are some deep breathing exercises to try:

1. **Abdominal Breathing**:
   - Find a comfortable seated or lying position.
   - Place one hand on your chest and the other on your abdomen.
   - Inhale deeply through your nose, allowing your abdomen to rise while keeping your chest relatively still.
   - Exhale slowly through your mouth, pulling your navel towards your spine.
   - Continue this pattern, focusing on the sensation of your abdomen rising and falling with each breath.

2. **4-7-8 Breathing**:
   - Sit or lie down in a comfortable position.
   - Close your eyes and take a deep breath in through your nose for a count of 4 seconds.
   - Hold your breath for a count of 7 seconds.
   - Exhale slowly and completely through your mouth, making a "whooshing" sound, for a count of 8 seconds.
   - Repeat this cycle for a few minutes, gradually working your way up to longer periods if comfortable.

3. **Equal Breathing**:
   - Sit comfortably and close your eyes.
   - Inhale through your nose for a count of 4 seconds.
   - Exhale through your nose for a count of 4 seconds.

- Continue this pattern, allowing the inhales and exhales to be of equal duration.

4. **Alternate Nostril Breathing**:
  - Sit comfortably with a straight spine.
  - Use your right thumb to close your right nostril and inhale through your left nostril for a count of 4 seconds.
  - Close your left nostril with your right ring finger, and release your right nostril as you exhale for a count of 4 seconds.
  - Inhale through your right nostril for a count of 4 seconds, close it with your thumb, and release your left nostril as you exhale for a count of 4 seconds.
  - Continue this pattern, focusing on the breath flowing through each nostril.

These deep breathing exercises are excellent for reducing stress, increasing relaxation, and promoting a sense of overall well-being. Practice them in a quiet, comfortable environment, and make it a part of your daily routine to maximize the benefits. Regular deep breathing can help you manage stress, improve your focus, and promote a greater sense of calm and balance in your life. Keep in mind that deep breathing can be beneficial anytime, anywhere, and can be used as a tool to ground yourself and find peace, no matter what challenges you may face during your day.

Day 5: Gentle Spinal Twists

Day 5 of the chair yoga practice introduces gentle spinal twists, which can be incredibly beneficial for releasing tension in the back, promoting flexibility, and improving overall spinal health.

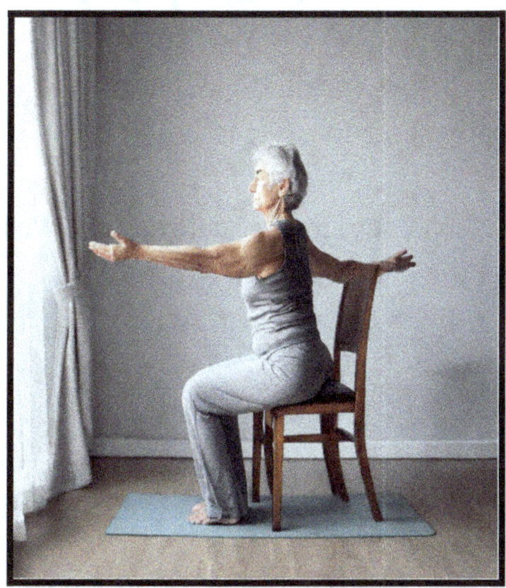

Begin by sitting comfortably in a sturdy chair with your feet planted firmly on the ground and your spine lengthened. Take a moment to connect with your breath, inhaling deeply through your nose and exhaling completely through your mouth to create a sense of relaxation and presence.

Here are some gentle spinal twists to incorporate into your chair yoga practice:

1. **Seated Twist**:

- Sit at the front edge of your chair, keeping your feet hip-width apart and your spine tall.

- Hold the sides of the chair seat and inhale as you lengthen your spine.

- Exhale as you gently rotate to the right, using your hands on the chair for support.

- Hold the twist for a few breaths, feeling the gentle stretch along your spine and the release of tension in your back.

- Inhale to return to the center, then exhale as you twist to the left, maintaining the length in your spine.

- Hold the twist for a few breaths before returning to the center.

2. Seated Eagle Twist:

- Sit with your feet firmly planted on the ground and your spine tall.

- Cross your right thigh over your left thigh and then place your right foot behind your left calf if comfortable. This is a modified seated version of the eagle pose.

- Place your left hand on your right knee, and your right hand on the back of the chair for support.

- Inhale to lengthen your spine, and exhale as you gently twist to the right.

- Hold the twist for a few breaths, feeling the release in your back, and then return to the center.

- Uncross your legs and repeat the twist on the other side, crossing your left thigh over your right and placing your left foot behind your right calf.

3. **Seated Cat-Cow Twist**:
- Sit comfortably in your chair with your feet flat on the ground and your hands resting on your knees.
- Inhale as you arch your back, lifting your chest and rolling your shoulders back (similar to cow pose in traditional yoga).
- Exhale as you round your back, tucking your chin to your chest and bringing your belly button towards your spine (similar to cat pose in traditional yoga).
- Continue to move through these seated cat-cow movements with your breath, adding a gentle twist to each side as you arch and round your back.

4. **Supported Spinal Twist:**
- Sit at the front edge of your chair with your feet planted firmly on the ground.
- Place your right hand on the back of the chair, and your left hand on the outside of your right thigh.
- Inhale to lengthen your spine, and exhale as you gently twist to the right, using the chair for support and avoiding any strain in your back.
- Hold the twist for a few breaths, feeling the gentle release in your spine, and then return to the center.

- Repeat the twist on the other side, placing your left hand on the back of the chair and your right hand on the outside of your left thigh.

Remember to move with mindfulness, paying attention to the sensations in your body and honoring its limits. These gentle spinal twists can help to relieve tension and promote flexibility, and they provide an opportunity to create space and mobility in your spine. As always, connect with your breath throughout the practice to cultivate a sense of calm and presence. Enjoy the benefits of gentle spinal twists as an integral part of your chair yoga journey, and feel the positive effects they bring to your body, mind, and spirit.

Day 6: Building Balance and Stability

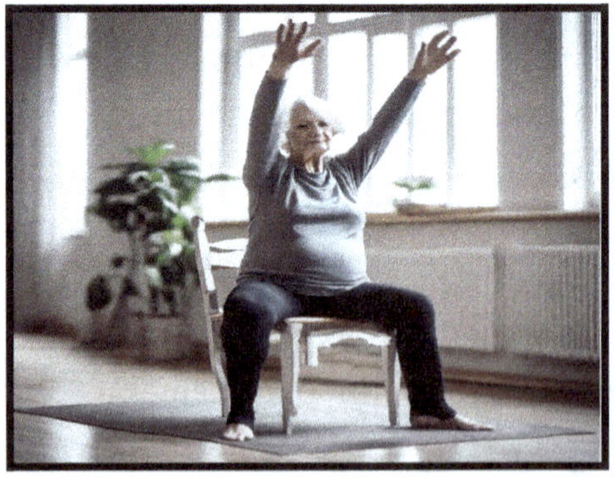

On Day 6 of your chair yoga practice, we'll focus on building balance and stability, which are essential for overall well-being and mobility. By incorporating these balance and stability exercises, you'll enhance your physical resilience and confidence. Here are some chair yoga movements to help improve your balance and stability:

1. **Seated Leg Extensions**:
   - Sit in your chair with your spine tall and your feet flat on the ground.
   - Hold onto the sides of the chair for support and lift your right foot a few inches off the ground, extending your leg straight out.
   - Hold for a few breaths, engaging your core for stability, and then lower your foot back down.
   - Switch to your left foot and repeat the extension.
   - For an added challenge, try extending both legs out one at a time, or even both legs simultaneously if comfortable, while maintaining a strong and upright posture.

2. **Seated Knee Lifts**:
   - Begin in the same seated position with your feet flat on the ground and your spine tall.
   - Hold onto the sides of the chair and lift your right knee towards your chest, engaging your core for stability.
   - Hold for a few breaths, feeling the activation in your hip flexors and lower abdominals, then lower your foot back down.

- Repeat the knee lift on your left side.

- For an additional challenge, you can alternate lifting your knees in a marching motion, focusing on maintaining your balance and stability as you move.

3. **Seated Side Leg Lifts**:

- Sit at the front edge of your chair with your feet hip-width apart and your spine tall.

- Hold onto the sides of the chair and extend your right leg out to the side, keeping it straight or slightly bent.

- Hold for a few breaths, feeling the engagement in your outer hip and thigh muscles, then lower your leg back down.

- Repeat the side leg lift with your left leg.

- To challenge yourself further, you can alternate lifting each leg to the side, focusing on controlled movements and balanced stability.

4. **Seated Spinal Balance**:

- Sit at the front edge of your chair with your feet flat on the ground and your spine tall.

- Extend your arms straight out in front of you at shoulder height, parallel to the ground.

- Engage your core muscles and slowly lean back, keeping your spine straight and your chest lifted, finding a point where you feel a comfortable challenge to your balance.

- Hold this position for a few breaths, then return to an upright seated position.

- Gradually increase the duration of the hold as your balance and stability improve.

5. **Seated Figure Four Stretch**:
- Sit with your spine tall and your feet flat on the ground.
- Cross your right ankle over your left knee, allowing your right knee to gently open to the side.
- Stay mindful of your posture and your breath as you feel a stretch in your outer hip and glute area.
- Hold the position for a few breaths, then release and repeat on the other side.

During these exercises, focus on maintaining steady, even breathing and concentrate on engaging your core muscles to assist in stabilizing your body. It's important to approach these movements with patience, listening to your body and recognizing your limits. Over time, with consistent practice, you may notice improvements in your balance, stability, and overall strength.

By incorporating these balance and stability-focused chair yoga exercises into your routine, you'll be nurturing your physical well-being and promoting a sense of groundedness in your everyday movements. Remember to approach these exercises with a sense of curiosity and joy, embracing the journey of cultivating balance and stability within your body.

Day 7: Relaxation and Mindfulness

On Day 7 of your chair yoga practice, the focus is on relaxation and mindfulness. This is a wonderful

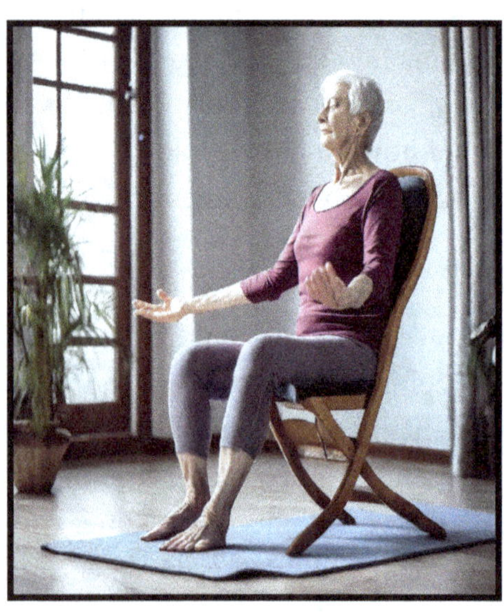

opportunity to cultivate a sense of calm and presence, promoting overall well-being and reducing stress. Here are some chair yoga movements and mindfulness practices to help you relax and center your mind:

1. **Deep Breathing Exercises**:

   - Begin by sitting comfortably in your chair with your feet flat on the ground and your spine tall.

   - Close your eyes and place your hands on your abdomen.

- Take a slow, deep breath in through your nose, feeling your abdomen rise as you fill your lungs with air.

- Exhale slowly and completely through your mouth, feeling your abdomen gently fall as you release the breath.

- Continue this deep breathing pattern for several breath cycles, focusing on the sensation of your breath moving in and out of your body. This practice helps calm the nervous system and increase a sense of relaxation.

2. **Seated Neck and Shoulder Stretches**:
   - Sit comfortably in your chair and allow your arms to rest by your sides.

   - Gently tilt your head to the right, bringing your right ear towards your right shoulder, and hold for a few breaths to feel a stretch along the left side of your neck. Repeat on the left side.

   - For shoulder stretches, inhale as you lift your shoulders up towards your ears, and exhale as you roll them back and down. Repeat this movement several times, releasing tension in the shoulders and upper back.

3. **Seated Forward Bend:**
   - Sit towards the front edge of your chair with your feet flat on the ground.

   - Inhale and lengthen your spine, then exhale as you hinge at your hips, leaning forward with a straight back.

- Allow your hands to rest on your shins, ankles, or the floor as you feel a gentle stretch in your lower back and the backs of your legs.

- Hold the forward bend for a few breaths, focusing on releasing tension and finding a sense of ease in the pose.

4. **Mindfulness Meditation**:

- Sit comfortably in your chair and close your eyes, bringing your attention to the present moment.

- Begin to notice the sensations in your body, the rise and fall of your breath, and the sounds around you without judgment.

- If your mind starts to wander, gently guide your focus back to your breath or a point of anchor, such as the feeling of your feet on the ground or the sensation of sitting in the chair.

- Practice being fully present in each moment, allowing a sense of serenity to envelop you.

Throughout these exercises, pay attention to your breath, body, and thoughts. Embrace a gentle and compassionate approach to your practice, honoring your body's needs and respecting your current limitations.

By incorporating relaxation techniques and mindfulness into your chair yoga practice, you'll nurture a deeper connection with yourself and promote a sense of inner peace. It's essential to approach these practices with an open heart and a willingness to be present in each moment. Celebrate the opportunity to cultivate relaxation and mindfulness in your daily routine, allowing these practices to support your overall well-being.

Week 2: Building Strength and Flexibility

During week 2 of your chair yoga practice, the focus shifts to building strength and flexibility, offering a

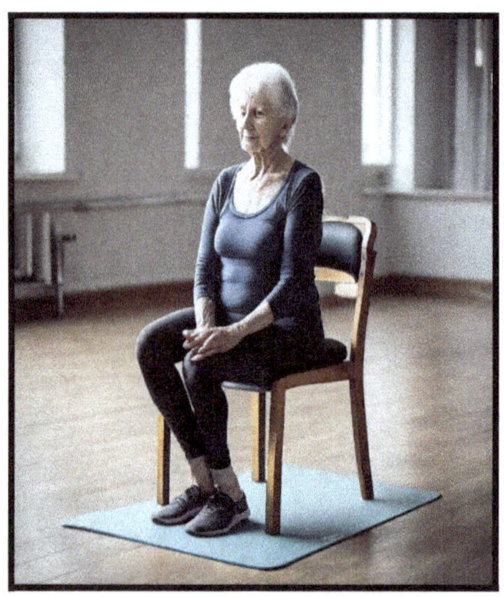

holistic approach to enhancing physical well-being. Each day's practice introduces specific movements tailored to target various aspects of your body, promoting strength, flexibility, and mindful awareness. Let's explore each day's focus:

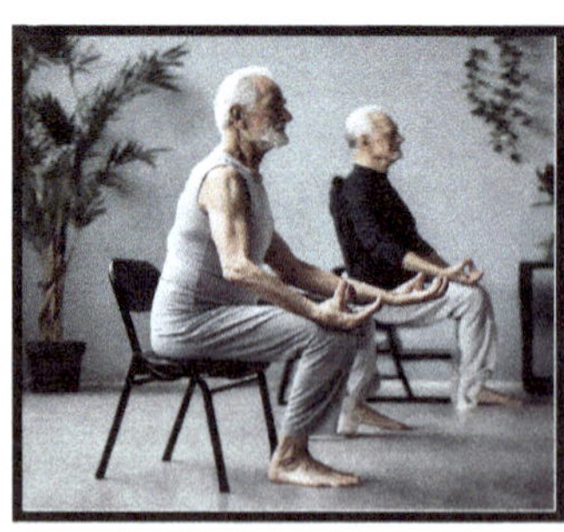

Day 8: Seated Side Stretches

On Day 8 of your chair yoga practice, the focus is on seated side stretches. Seated side stretches are a wonderful way to increase flexibility in the side body, alleviate tension, and promote a sense of openness. Here's a brief guide to help you engage in seated side stretches effectively:

1. **Find a Comfortable Seated Position**: Sit comfortably on a sturdy chair with your feet flat on the ground and your spine tall. Ensure that you are sitting with proper alignment, and feel your sitting bones grounding into the chair.

2. **Lengthen Your Spine**: Inhale and lengthen your spine, imagining your head reaching toward the ceiling. This allows for optimal posture and alignment throughout the stretches.

3. **Gentle Side Bend to the Right**: As you exhale, slowly and gently side bend to the right, bringing your right hand to the side of the chair seat or armrest. Extend your left arm over your head, reaching toward the right side to deepen the stretch.

4. **Feel the Stretch**: Focus on feeling a gentle stretch along the left side of your body as you hold the pose for several breaths. Be mindful of not straining and only going as far as is comfortable for you.

5. **Gentle Side Bend to the Left:** Inhale as you return to an upright seated position, then repeat the side bend to the left, mirroring the movement and stretch on the opposite side.

6. **Breathe Mindfully**: Throughout the stretches, maintain a steady and soothing breath, allowing your exhalations to assist in deepening the stretch and releasing tension.

7. **Gradually Release**: After holding the stretches on both sides, return to a neutral seated position, taking a moment to acknowledge any sensations in your body.

Remember that the breath is essential in chair yoga, so continue to synchronize your movements with your breath, fostering a harmonious connection between body and breath. As always, listen to your body, and modify the stretches as needed to suit your individual range of motion and comfort. Seated side stretches are a gentle and effective way to promote flexibility and release tension in the side body, so embrace the opportunity to explore these movements mindfully and with awareness.

Day 9: Strengthening the Core

On Day 9 of your chair yoga practice, the focus is on strengthening the core. Engaging in chair yoga exercises that target the core muscles can support stability, promote better posture, and contribute to overall strength. Here's a tailored approach for incorporating core-strengthening movements into your chair yoga practice:

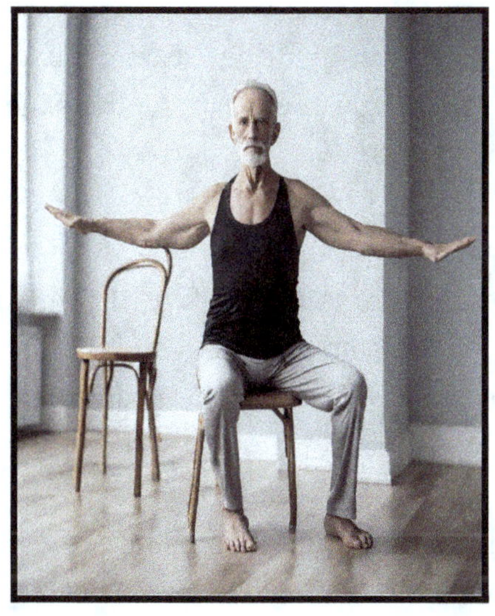

1. **Seated Posture Awareness:** Begin by sitting comfortably on your chair, ensuring that your feet are grounded and your spine is tall. Center your awareness on your breath, allowing for a few moments to connect with your internal rhythm.

2. **Seated Cat-Cow Movements**: Initiate the core-strengthening practice with gentle seated cat-cow movements. As you inhale, arch your back slightly, allowing your belly to come forward and your chest to open. Upon exhaling, round your back, drawing your

belly button in towards your spine. Repeat this movement, synchronizing breath with movement, to engage and awaken the core muscles.

3. **Seated Knee Lifts**: While maintaining an upright seated position, lift one knee towards your chest and hold for a few breaths, engaging your core to support the movement. Alternate between lifting each knee, maintaining a smooth and steady breath throughout the exercise.

4. **Seated Spinal Twists**: Engage in gentle seated spinal twists to further engage the core muscles. Twist towards one side, using the support of the chair as you hold the twist and breathe consciously. Return to center and repeat the twist on the opposite side.

5. **Breath-Centric Engagement**: Throughout these core-strengthening movements, maintain a focus on deep, diaphragmatic breathing. Allow your breath to flow naturally and support the engagement of your core muscles, fostering a mindful integration of breath and movement.

6. **Mindful Conclusion**: Conclude the core-strengthening sequence with a few moments of seated relaxation, acknowledging the sensations in your body and the subtle activation in your core.

Remember to honor your body's limits and modify the movements as needed to suit your comfort and ability. The core-strengthening practice in chair yoga serves as an opportunity to cultivate stability and presence, enabling you to establish a deeper connection to your body's center. Embrace this practice with mindful attention and a commitment to nurturing your core strength as an integral part of your chair yoga journey.

Day 10: Leg Strengthening Exercises

On Day 10 of your chair yoga practice, the focus is on leg strengthening exercises. Strengthening the legs

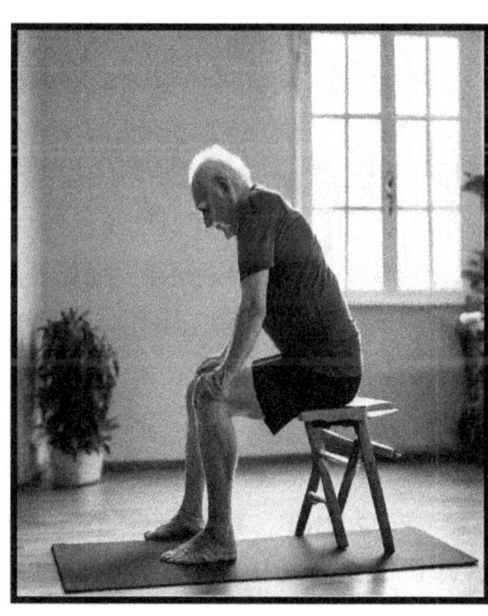

through chair yoga movements can help improve stability, balance, and overall lower body strength. Here's a tailored approach to incorporate leg-strengthening exercises into your chair yoga practice:

1. **Seated Mountain Pose**: Begin by sitting tall in your chair with your feet flat on the floor, hip-width apart. Press your feet into the ground, engaging the muscles in your legs as if you were standing in mountain pose. Feel a gentle lift in your pelvic floor and spine as you ground through your feet.

2. **Seated Knee Extensions:** Lift one foot slightly off the floor and extend your leg in front of you. Hold the extended position for a few breaths, feeling the engagement in your quadriceps and calf muscles. Lower the foot back to the floor and repeat with the other leg.

3. **Seated Leg Lifts**: Keeping your posture tall and your core engaged, lift one leg straight out in front of you, parallel to the floor. Hold for a few breaths, keeping the thigh engaged. Lower the leg and repeat on the other side.

4. **Seated Heel Raises**: Place your hands on your thighs for support and lift your heels off the ground, pressing the balls of your feet into the floor. Feel the engagement in your calf muscles as you hold the position for a few breaths. Lower your heels back to the ground and repeat the movement.

5. **Seated Warrior Pose Variation**: Extend one leg straight out to the side, with the heel on the floor and

toes pointing up. Press into the outer edge of your foot, engaging the muscles in your outer thigh. Hold for several breaths before releasing and repeating on the other side.

6. **Breath and Mindfulness**: Throughout these leg-strengthening exercises, maintain deep, mindful breathing, allowing your breath to support and complement the movements. Stay focused on your body's sensations and the engagement of your leg muscles.

7. **Seated Relaxation**: After completing the leg-strengthening sequence, take a moment to sit with your eyes closed, breathing deeply, and appreciating the effort and attention you've devoted to your leg muscles.

As always, listen to your body and modify the movements as needed to ensure comfort and safety. Embrace the opportunity to cultivate strength and stability in your lower body through these chair yoga exercises, fostering a deeper connection to your legs and overall well-being.

Day 11: Chair Warrior Poses

On Day 11 of your chair yoga practice, the focus is on exploring chair warrior poses. Warrior poses are known for building strength, stability, and confidence. Adapting them to a chair yoga practice allows you to experience the benefits of these empowering poses while seated. Here's a tailored approach to incorporate chair warrior poses into your practice:

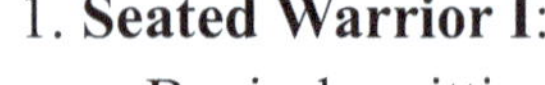

1. **Seated Warrior I:**
   - Begin by sitting in your chair with your spine tall and your feet grounded.
   - Extend one leg back, keeping the foot flat on the floor. Your other leg should be bent at a 90-degree angle, with the knee aligned over the ankle.
   - Raise your arms overhead, stretching upward to feel the lengthening of your spine.
   - Hold the pose for several breaths, feeling the strength and stability it brings to your body.

2. **Seated Warrior II**:

- From Seated Warrior I, open your hips and shoulders to the side of your extended leg.

- Extend your arms out to the sides, parallel to the floor, with your gaze focused over your front hand.

- Feel the grounded stability of your lower body while reaching outward through your fingertips.

3. **Seated Warrior III**:

- Sit toward the front edge of your chair, extending one leg straight out in front of you.

- Hinge forward from your hips, reaching your arms forward while lifting your back leg off the ground, parallel to the floor.

- Engage your core for balance and stability, feeling the strength and focus in your entire body.

Throughout these chair warrior poses, maintain deep, mindful breathing, allowing your breath to support and complement the movements. Embrace the sense of empowerment and strength that these poses offer, even from a seated position.

As always, listen to your body and modify the poses as needed to ensure comfort and safety. Allow the chair warrior poses to bring a sense of confidence, inner strength, and mindfulness to your chair yoga practice.

Each breath and movement can contribute to a deeper connection to your body and a renewed sense of well-being.

Day 12: Hip Openers

On Day 12 of your chair yoga practice, the focus is on exploring hip-opening exercises. Hip openers can

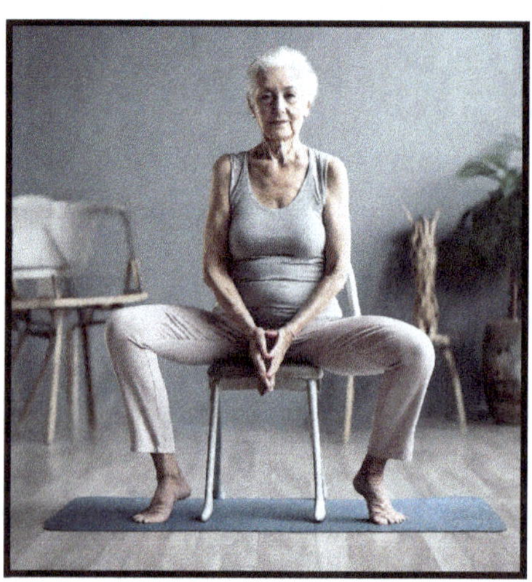

help improve flexibility, mobility, and overall comfort in your hips and lower body. Here's a tailored approach to incorporate hip-opening exercises into your chair yoga practice:

1. **Seated Hip Circles**:
   - Begin by sitting tall in your chair with your feet flat on the floor and your hands resting on your thighs.
   - Slowly begin to circle your hips in one direction, focusing on creating smooth, gentle movements. Allow

your breath to guide the motion, letting it flow naturally with each circle.

- After several rotations, reverse the direction of your circles to balance the movement.

2. **Seated Pigeon Pose**:

- Sit toward the front edge of your chair and cross one ankle over the opposite knee, creating a figure-four shape with your legs.

- Gently press down on the crossed knee to feel a comfortable stretch in the outer hip of the crossed leg.

- Sit tall and breathe deeply, allowing the stretch to gradually release any tension in your hips.

3. **Seated Knee to Chest Stretch**:

- While seated, hug one knee into your chest, interlacing your fingers around your shin.

- Feel the gentle opening in your hip as you draw the knee closer to your chest, breathing deeply into the sensation.

- Release the leg and switch to the other side, repeating the stretch for both hips.

4. **Seated Figure-Four Stretch**:

- Sit tall in your chair and cross one ankle over the opposite knee, similar to the position in Seated Pigeon Pose.

- Maintain a tall spine as you gently hinge forward at your hips, feeling a stretch in the crossed hip.

- Breathe into the stretch and find a comfortable depth that allows for a gentle release in the hip.

5. **Seated Bound Angle Pose**:

- Sit toward the front edge of your chair and bring the soles of your feet together, allowing your knees to open outward.

- Hold onto your ankles or shins and gently press your thighs down, feeling a comfortable opening in your hips and inner thighs.

- Breathe deeply, allowing the pose to create space and ease in your hips.

Throughout these hip-opening exercises, maintain deep, mindful breathing, allowing your breath to support and complement the movements. Embrace the opportunity to nurture flexibility and mobility in your hips and lower body, fostering a deeper connection to your body and overall well-being.

As always, listen to your body and modify the exercises as needed to ensure comfort and safety. Embrace the sense of release and freedom that these hip openers bring to your chair yoga practice, allowing each breath to guide you toward greater comfort and ease in your hips.

Day 13: Gentle Backbends

For Day 13 of your chair yoga practice, the focus is on gentle backbends to promote spinal mobility and openness. Incorporating gentle backbends can help

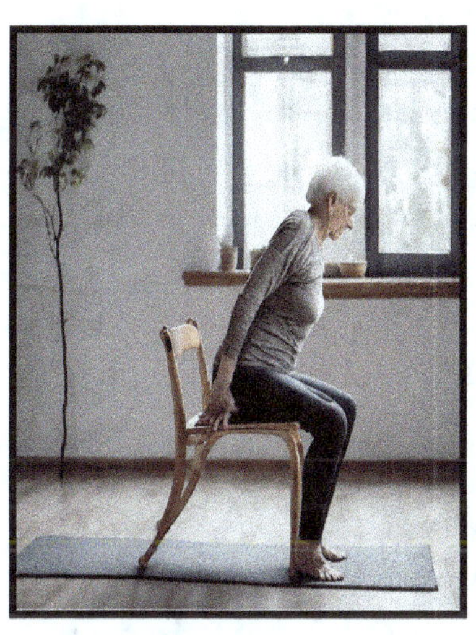

alleviate tension, improve posture, and enhance overall flexibility. Here's a tailored approach to integrate gentle backbends into your chair yoga routine:

1. **Seated Cat-Cow Stretch**:

- Begin by sitting tall in your chair with your hands resting on your thighs.

- As you inhale, arch your back and lift your chest, gently gazing upward (Cow Pose).

- As you exhale, round your spine, tucking your chin to your chest (Cat Pose).

- Flow between these two movements, synchronizing your breath with the movement of your spine, allowing each transition to be smooth and fluid.

2. Seated Backbend with Arm Reach:
- Sit toward the front edge of your chair, grounding your feet onto the floor.
- Interlace your fingers behind your back, gently pressing your palms together.
- As you inhale, lift your chest and extend your arms, allowing your gaze to lift upward if comfortable.
- Maintain a gentle, steady arch in your upper back, feeling a comfortable stretch across the front of your chest and shoulders.
- Release the pose with an exhale and repeat as desired, finding a rhythm that feels supportive and spacious for your back.

3. Supported Seated Backbend:
- Sit comfortably toward the front of your chair, placing your hands on the sides of the seat for support.
- As you inhale, gently arch your back, lifting your heart and chest upward, while keeping your hands grounded for stability.
- Focus on creating length through your spine, feeling a pleasant stretch across the front of your body without straining.

- Breathe deeply into the gentle extension, allowing your breath to foster a sense of ease and openness in your back.

4. Seated Heart Opener:
- Sit tall with your hands resting on your thighs.
- As you inhale, lift your sternum and gently draw your shoulder blades together, allowing your chest to open.
- Keep your chin parallel to the ground, maintaining a comfortable extension through the upper back and chest.
- Exhale and release the pose, repeating as needed to invite a sense of spaciousness and freedom in your upper body.

5. Seated Extended Camel Pose:
- Sit toward the front edge of your chair, grounding your feet firmly onto the floor.
- Place your hands on your lower back for support as you gently lean back, allowing your heart to lift and your gaze to reach upward if comfortable.
- Find a gentle arch in your upper back, maintaining support through your legs and core.
- Breathe deeply as you hold the pose, nurturing a sense of openness and expansiveness in your back.

Throughout these gentle backbends, remain attentive to your breath, allowing it to guide the movement of your spine and foster a sense of relaxation and spaciousness.

Approach each posture with awareness and gentleness, honoring the unique needs of your body.

Remember to modify the exercises as necessary to ensure comfort and safety. Embrace the opportunity to cultivate mobility, openness, and ease in your back, allowing each gentle backbend to create a pathway for greater comfort and well-being.

Day 14: Relaxation and Mindfulness

Welcome to Day 14 of your chair yoga practice, where the focus is on relaxation and mindfulness. Cultivating a sense of calm and presence can have profound effects on your overall well-being. Here's a tailored approach to integrate relaxation and mindfulness techniques into your chair yoga routine:

1. **Seated Deep Breathing**:
   - Sit comfortably with your feet grounded on the floor and your hands resting on your thighs.
   - Close your eyes if comfortable, and take a few moments to settle into stillness.
   - Begin to deepen your breath, focusing on inhaling through your nose and exhaling through your mouth.

- With each inhalation, envision a sense of calm and ease filling your body, and with each exhalation, release any tension or stress.

2. Seated Mindful Body Scan:
- Start by bringing your attention to your feet. Notice any sensations, such as warmth, tingling, or pressure.
- Gradually shift your awareness up through your legs, hips, abdomen, chest, back, shoulders, arms, and hands, observing each part of your body with curiosity and acceptance.
- Pay attention to any areas of tension or discomfort, and with each exhalation, imagine those areas softening and releasing.
- Complete the body scan by bringing your focus to your head and face, allowing any tension in these areas to melt away.

3. Seated Neck and Shoulder Rolls:
- Inhale as you gently roll your shoulders up towards your ears.
- Exhale as you roll them back and down, allowing any tension to release.
- Continue this movement, allowing your breath to guide the pace and rhythm of the rolls.
- After a few repetitions, reverse the direction, rolling your shoulders forward and up on the inhale, and back and down on the exhale.

4. **Seated Forward Fold:**

- Sit forward in your chair, with your feet firmly planted on the ground.

- As you inhale, lengthen your spine, and as you exhale, gently hinge forward from your hips, allowing your chest to approach your thighs.

- Let your arms hang loosely or reach for your shins or the floor, finding a position that feels comfortable for your body.

- Breathe deeply into your back body, allowing your breath to create space and relaxation in the muscles of your back.

5. **Seated Meditation**:

- Sit comfortably, with your spine tall and your hands resting on your lap or knees.

- Close your eyes if it feels right for you, or soften your gaze.

- Begin to focus on your breath, allowing your inhales and exhales to anchor you in the present moment.

- If your mind starts to wander, gently guide your focus back to your breath without judgment.

Throughout these relaxation and mindfulness practices, let go of any expectations and simply allow yourself to be present and compassionate toward yourself. Use your breath as a tool to ground and center yourself, fostering a sense of tranquility and ease.

By integrating these techniques into your chair yoga routine, you can harness the power of relaxation and mindfulness to support your overall well-being, both on and off the chair. Embrace this opportunity to nurture a deeper connection with yourself, cultivating a sense of peace and serenity in your daily life.

Week 3: Enhancing Mobility and Balance

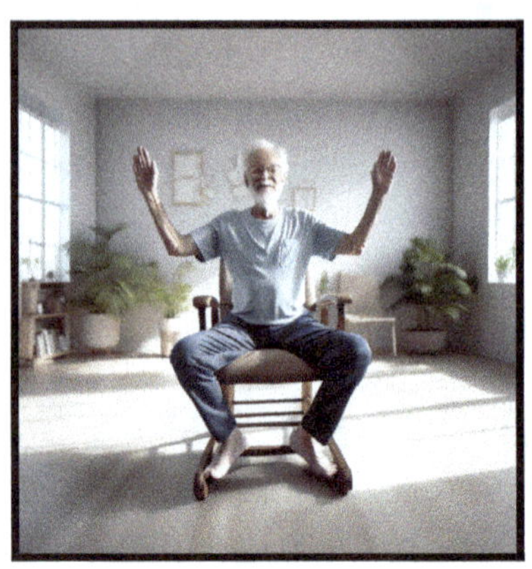

Week 3 of your chair yoga practice focuses on enhancing mobility and balance. These chair yoga sessions are designed to improve your range of motion, strengthen your muscles, and promote stability. Let's break down each day's practice:

Day 15: Seated Mountain Pose

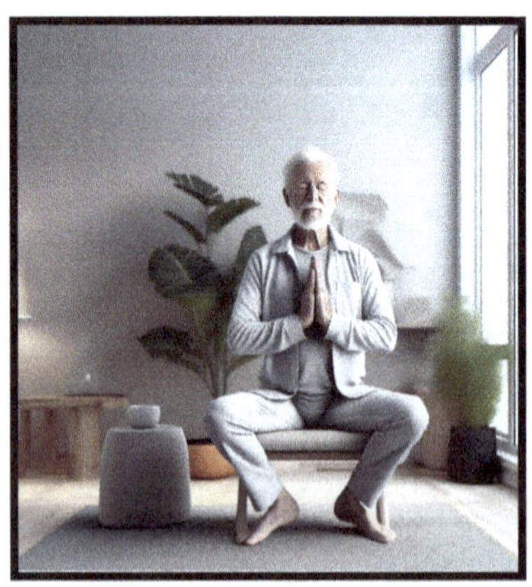

Seated Mountain Pose is a foundational chair yoga posture that focuses on grounding, elongating the spine, and promoting a sense of stability and mindfulness. Here's a step-by-step guide to practicing Seated Mountain Pose:

1. Start by sitting tall in your chair with your feet flat on the ground and your hands resting on your thighs or knees.

2. Take a moment to find your sit bones firmly rooted into the chair, creating a stable foundation for your seated position.

3. Close your eyes or maintain a soft gaze, allowing your breath to become steady and even.

4. On an inhalation, extend your arms out to the sides and reach them overhead, palms facing each other or touching.

5. As you reach your arms up, lengthen your spine, imagining that you are growing taller with each breath.

6. Keep your shoulders relaxed and away from your ears as you extend upward.

7. Exhale and slowly bring your hands back down to your heart center, maintaining an awareness of your breath and body throughout the movement.

8. Repeat this movement, synchronizing your breath with the flow of your arms. Inhale as you reach up, and exhale as you bring your hands back to your heart center.

Practicing Seated Mountain Pose can help you cultivate a sense of presence, stability, and mindfulness in your chair yoga practice. It also provides an opportunity to focus on your breath and physical alignment while seated, promoting a deep sense of grounding and balance.

Day 16: Improving Range of Motion in the Arms

On day 16 of the chair yoga practice plan, we will

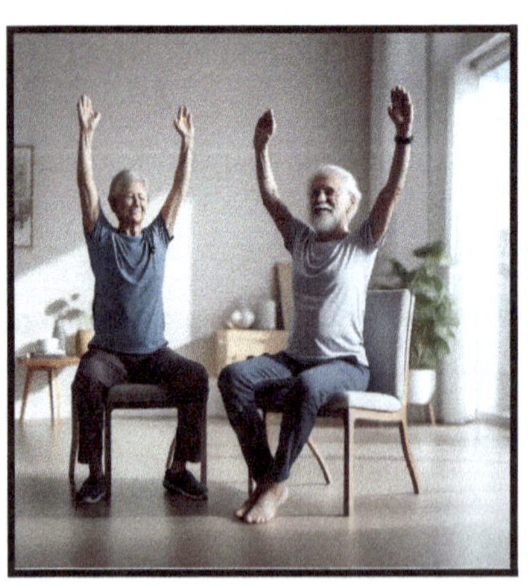

focus on improving the range of motion in the arms. This sequence will help increase flexibility and mobility in the shoulders, elbows, and wrists, leading to enhanced functional movement and a sense of ease in daily activities. Below are some chair yoga exercises to achieve this:

1. **Seated Arm Circles**:
   - Start by sitting in a comfortable and upright position.
   - Extend your arms out to the sides at shoulder height.
   - Begin to make slow and controlled circular motions with your arms, moving through a full range of motion.
   - Gradually increase the size of the circles, feeling the stretch and engagement in your shoulders and arms.
   - After several repetitions, reverse the direction of the circles.
   - Focus on maintaining smooth and steady breathing throughout the movement.

2. **Eagle Arms**:
   - Sit tall in your chair with your feet grounded.
   - Stretch your arms out in front of you at shoulder height.
   - Cross your right arm over the left, bringing your palms together if possible, or simply holding onto your shoulders.
   - Lift your elbows slightly as you draw your shoulders down, feeling a stretch across your upper back and shoulders.
   - Hold the position for a few breaths, then release and repeat with the left arm crossing over the right.

3. **Wrist Flexor and Extensor Stretch**:

- Extend your right arm out in front of you, palm facing down.

- Use your left hand to gently press down on the fingers of your right hand, stretching the wrist and forearm.

- After holding for a few breaths, switch to the other hand, this time with the palm facing up, and gently press the fingers back toward the body to stretch the wrist flexors.

4. **Cow Face Arms**:

- Extend your right arm up toward the ceiling and bend your elbow, reaching your hand down your upper back.

- Use your left hand to reach behind your back and try to clasp your fingers together, or use a strap or towel to connect your hands if they don't reach.

- Feel the stretch in your triceps and shoulders as you gently draw your elbows in opposite directions.

- Hold for a few breaths, then release and switch arms.

These exercises are designed to gently and effectively improve the range of motion in your arms, shoulders, and wrists. Consistently practicing these movements will help enhance flexibility and mobility, reducing stiffness and promoting a greater sense of comfort and ease in your upper body. Always remember to move within your comfortable range of motion and breathe steadily as you perform these exercises.

Day 17: Gentle Chair Twist Variations

On day 17 of the chair yoga practice plan, we will focus

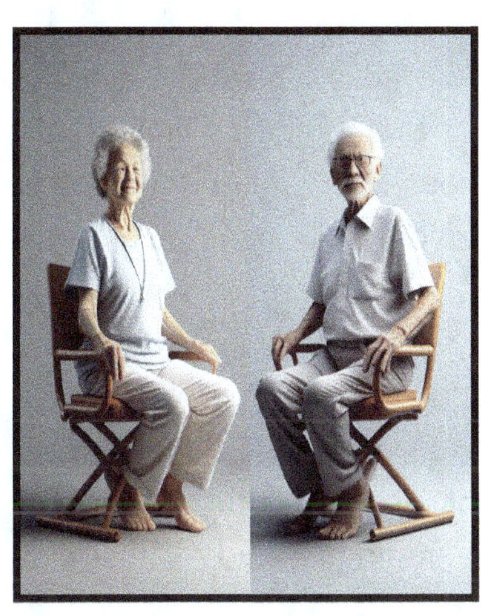

on gentle chair twist variations to promote spinal mobility, release tension, and improve overall flexibility. Twists help to massage the internal organs, stimulate digestion, and promote a sense of relaxation. Here are some chair yoga variations for gentle twists:

1. **Seated Twist**:

- Sit in a comfortable and upright position with your feet flat on the ground.

- Inhale as you lengthen through your spine, and as you exhale, gently twist to the right, placing your left hand on the outside of your right thigh and your right hand on the back of the chair.

- Keep your gaze soft and steady, looking over your right shoulder if it's comfortable for your neck.

- With each inhalation, find a little more length through your spine, and with each exhalation, deepen the twist if it feels appropriate for your body.

- Hold the twist for several breaths, then slowly release and repeat on the other side.

2. **Chest Opener Twist**:
   - Start by sitting tall in your chair.
   - Extend your arms out to the sides at shoulder height.
   - Inhale to lengthen your spine, and as you exhale, twist to the right, crossing your left hand over the top of your right thigh and placing your right hand on the back of the chair.
   - As you settle into the twist, open through your chest and shoulders, gently pressing your left arm into your right thigh to deepen the stretch.
   - Feel the twist from the base of your spine all the way up to your neck, maintaining steady breathing throughout.
   - After holding the twist, return to the center and repeat on the opposite side.

3. **Seated Eagle Twist**:
   - Start by sitting tall in your chair and extend your arms out to the sides at shoulder height.

- Cross your right arm under your left, bringing your palms together if possible, or simply hugging your shoulders.

- Inhale to lengthen your spine, and as you exhale, twist to the right, hooking your left elbow on the outside of your right thigh.

- Press your palms or forearms together to deepen the twist while keeping your shoulders relaxed and down.

- Maintain the twist for a few breaths, then gently release and repeat on the other side.

4. **Seated Half Lord of the Fishes Twist**:

- Begin in a seated position with your legs extended in front of you.

- Bend your right knee and cross it over your left leg, placing your right foot on the ground outside your left thigh.

- Inhale to lengthen through your spine, and as you exhale, twist to the right, using your left elbow to hug your right knee and your right hand on the seat or back of the chair for support.

- Gaze over your right shoulder, feeling the length through your spine and the gentle twist in your torso.

- Hold the twist for several breaths, then slowly release and switch to the other side.

These chair yoga twist variations offer a gentle way to promote spinal mobility and release tension throughout the torso while seated. When practicing these variations, focus on moving with awareness, maintaining steady breathing, and respecting your body's natural limitations. Twists can offer a refreshing release for the spine and provide a sense of rejuvenation and relaxation.

Day 18: Chair Side Plank and Leg Lifts

On day 18 of the chair yoga practice plan, we will incorporate chair side plank and leg lifts to strengthen

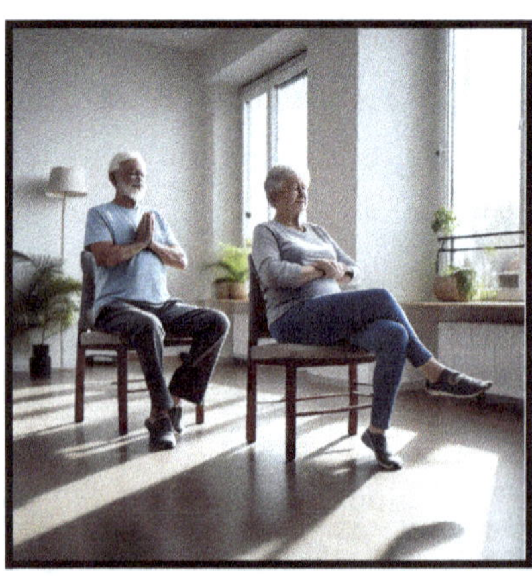

the core, improve balance, and engage the lower body muscles. These movements can be beneficial for building stability and promoting better posture. Here's how to practice chair side plank and leg lifts:

Chair Side Plank:

1. Begin by sitting on the edge of the chair with your feet flat on the ground, hip-width apart.

2. Place your right hand on the seat of the chair, slightly behind your hip, and press into the hand to lift your hips off the chair, coming into a side plank position.

3. Extend your legs long, keeping your body in a straight line from head to heels. Your left arm can be extended toward the ceiling or placed on your hip for support.

4. Engage your core muscles, and maintain a steady breath as you hold the side plank for several breath cycles.

5. Slowly lower your hips back to the chair, then switch to the other side and repeat the process.

Chair Leg Lifts:

1. Sit tall on the chair with your hands resting on the sides for support.

2. Engage your abdominal muscles and lift one leg straight out in front of you, parallel to the ground.

3. Hold the lifted leg for a few breaths, maintaining an upright posture and focusing on engaging the core and leg muscles.

4. Lower the leg back down and repeat on the opposite side.

5. For an added challenge, you can alternate lifting the legs or hold each leg lift for a longer duration.

Tips *for Practicing Chair Side Plank and Leg Lifts:*

- **Focus on alignment:** Keep your body in a straight line during chair side plank, and ensure that your lifted leg is parallel to the ground during leg lifts.
- **Use the chair for support**: If needed, you can place your bottom hand on the chair seat for added stability during side plank, and use your hands for support during leg lifts.
- **Mindful breathing**: Maintain steady, mindful breathing throughout the movements to enhance focus and relaxation.

These chair yoga movements provide a creative way to incorporate core and lower body strengthening exercises while seated. As with any physical activity, it's essential to listen to your body, move within your comfort level, and make any necessary modifications to support your individual needs. These exercises can contribute to overall strength, balance, and stability, offering a holistic approach to chair yoga practice.

Day 19: Chair Tree Pose

On day 19 of the chair yoga practice plan, we will incorporate the Chair Tree Pose to enhance balance,

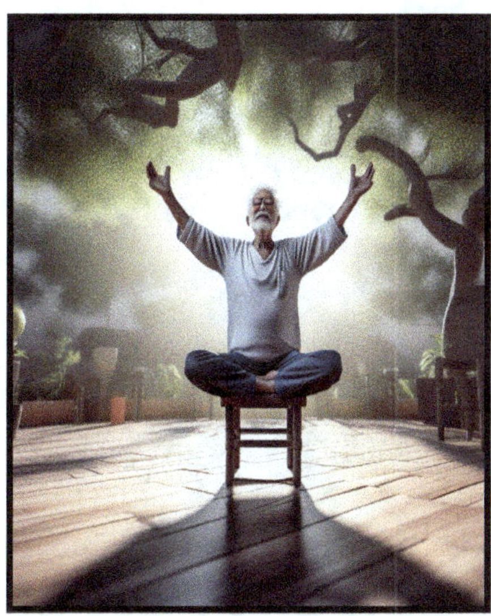

stability, and focus. Chair Tree Pose is a modified version of the traditional Tree Pose, allowing individuals to experience the benefits of the posture while being supported by the chair. Here's how to practice Chair Tree Pose:

1. Begin by sitting tall on the chair, with your feet flat on the ground and your spine comfortably aligned.
2. Engage your core muscles and maintain a steady, grounding connection with the chair and the floor.
3. Shift your weight slightly onto your left foot while keeping the right foot grounded.
4. Slowly lift your right foot off the ground and place the sole of the right foot against the inside of the left calf or inner thigh, depending on your comfort and balance.

5. Avoid placing the foot directly against the knee joint to prevent excessive pressure on the joint.

6. Find a focal point in front of you to help maintain balance and stability.

7. Bring your palms together at heart center or extend your arms overhead in a modified variation of the traditional Tree Pose.

8. Hold the position, maintaining steady breathing and a sense of rootedness through the supporting foot.

Benefits of Chair Tree Pose:

- Balance and Stability: Practicing Chair Tree Pose helps improve balance and stability by engaging the muscles of the standing leg and promoting a steady, grounded connection with the floor.

- Concentration and Focus: The focus required to maintain the pose can help enhance mental concentration and mindfulness.

- Lower Body Strength: The leg and foot muscles are engaged and strengthened as they support the body's weight in the pose, contributing to lower body stability.

Tips for Practicing Chair Tree Pose:

- **Use the chair for support**: The chair provides a supportive prop for maintaining balance and stability while practicing the pose.

- **Explore variations**: You can modify the position of the lifted foot to find the most comfortable and sustainable variation for your body.
- **Gentle engagement**: Avoid forcing the lifted foot too high up the standing leg to prevent strain. Focus on finding a position that allows you to maintain balance without compromising comfort.

Chair Tree Pose is a wonderful way to integrate a standing balance posture into a seated practice, offering the benefits of improved balance and stability while respecting individual comfort and mobility levels. As with any yoga practice, it's important to approach the pose with mindful awareness, honor your body's limitations, and make any necessary adjustments to ensure a safe and enjoyable experience.

Adding Chair Tree Pose to your chair yoga routine can provide a refreshing opportunity to explore balance and focus, offering a unique blend of seated and standing elements within a supportive framework. As always, remember to practice with awareness, listen to your body, and enjoy the journey of mindful movement.

Day 20: Building Balance and Stability

Day 20 of the chair yoga practice plan will focus on further building balance and stability through a series of

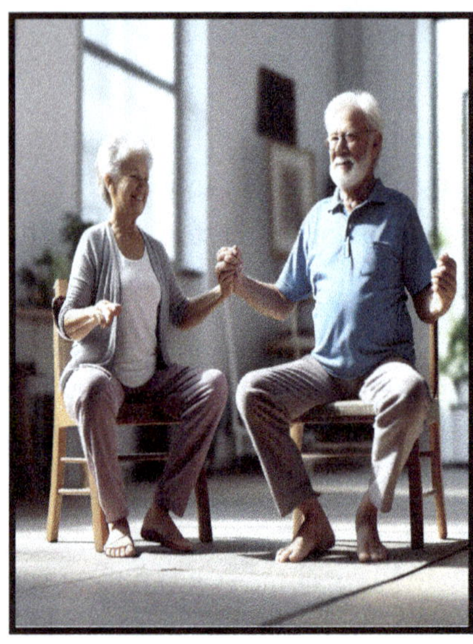

seated and standing poses. Developing these foundational attributes is essential for enhancing overall well-being and mobility. The sequence for Day 20 will include a combination of chair-assisted and standing balance poses to cater to a range of abilities and preferences.

Here's an outline for Day 20's practice:

1. **Seated Mountain Pose**: Begin the session with Seated Mountain Pose to ground yourself, center your focus, and establish a strong, stable posture while seated in the chair. This will prepare your mind and body for the balance-focused sequence.

2. **Seated Side Stretch:** Transition into a gentle seated side stretch to awaken the sides of the body, encourage openness in the ribcage, and prepare for the upcoming balance poses.

3. **Chair-assisted Half Moon Pose:** Use the chair for support while transitioning into a modified Half Moon Pose. This variation enables you to focus on balance and stability without compromising safety and support.

4. **Seated Spinal Twist:** Re-engage with a seated spinal twist to release tension, re-center your energy, and maintain flexibility in the spine.

5. **Chair Tree Pose:** Revisit the Chair Tree Pose to solidify your balance and stability practice. Explore the pose with a deeper sense of concentration and steadiness.

6. **Chair-assisted Warrior III:** Utilize the chair for stability and support as you incorporate a modified version of Warrior III. This pose will further challenge your balance and strength while respecting your individual capabilities.

7. **Seated Forward Fold:** Conclude the sequence with a seated forward fold to release any accumulated tension while maintaining a focus on stability and grounding.

This sequence aims to provide a comprehensive balance and stability-building experience by incorporating both seated and standing positions. The chair acts as a supportive tool throughout the practice, ensuring accessibility and safety for individuals with varying mobility levels.

By consistently nurturing balance and stability, practitioners can enhance their physical and mental well-being. These attributes are vital for everyday activities and contribute to a sense of confidence and body awareness. Additionally, the mindfulness cultivated during balance-focused practices can have a positive impact on mental clarity and emotional equilibrium.

As you embark on Day 20's balance and stability practice, remember to approach each pose with an open mind, focusing on the journey of self-discovery and growth. Embrace the support of the chair as you explore the nuances of balance and stability, and always listen to your body's cues to ensure a safe and enjoyable practice.

Day 21: Relaxation and Mindfulness

Day 21 of the chair yoga practice plan will center around relaxation and mindfulness, providing an

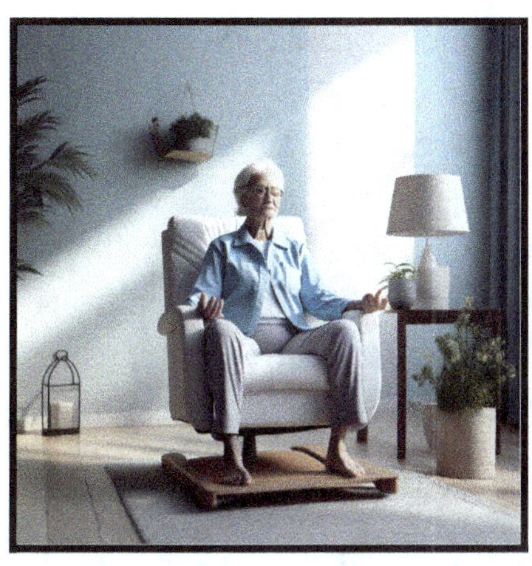

opportunity to unwind, release tension, and cultivate a sense of inner calm. This session is designed to promote mental and emotional well-being, making it an essential component of a holistic yoga practice.

Here's a curated sequence for Day 21 focusing on relaxation and mindfulness:

1. **Seated Heart Opener**: Begin the session with a gentle seated heart opener to invite a sense of openness and receptivity. As you draw back your shoulders and lift your heart, focus on inviting relaxation into your body and mind.

2. **Seated Cat-Cow Stretch**: Transition into a flowing seated Cat-Cow stretch to encourage spinal mobility, release tension, and synchronize breath with movement. Emphasize the gentle undulation of the spine to promote a sense of ease and relaxation.

3. **Seated Forward Fold**: Engage in a seated forward fold to encourage introspection and release any lingering physical or mental tension. With each breath, allow yourself to soften into the posture and let go of stress.

4. **Seated Pigeon Pose:** Explore a seated variation of Pigeon Pose to release tension in the hips and cultivate a sense of emotional release and surrender. Embrace mindfulness as you breathe into any areas of tightness or resistance.

5. **Seated Twist**: Revisit a seated twist to unwind the spine and promote a sense of detoxification and rejuvenation. Focus on the gentle rotation while maintaining a calm and centered mind.

6. **Guided Meditation**: Transition into a guided meditation, perhaps focusing on a relaxation technique, visualization, or breath awareness. Allow this time for deep relaxation and mental rejuvenation.

7. **Final Relaxation**: Conclude the practice with a period of deep relaxation or Savasana. Utilize supportive props such as a blanket or cushion to enhance comfort and encourage a profound sense of letting go.

Throughout this session, emphasize the cultivation of mindfulness, allowing yourself to fully engage in the present moment with a non-judgmental awareness. Embrace the opportunity to let go of distractions and external stressors, directing your attention inward to nurture your mental and emotional well-being.

By dedicating time to relaxation and mindfulness, practitioners can experience a sense of renewal, reduce stress, and enhance overall mental clarity and emotional balance. This practice creates space for self-reflection and inner exploration, fostering a deeper connection with oneself and promoting a profound sense of tranquility.

As you engage in Day 21's relaxation and mindfulness practice, embrace this opportunity to nurture your inner landscape, fostering a state of calm and presence. Allow the practice to serve as a sanctuary, providing a respite from the demands of daily life and empowering you to cultivate a greater sense of well-being. Remember to approach this session with an open heart and a willingness to surrender to the experience, honoring your personal journey toward relaxation and mindfulness.

Week 4: Putting It All Together

Week 4 of the chair yoga practice plan provides a diverse and comprehensive approach to integrating the key elements of chair yoga, including full-body movement, traditional yoga sequences adapted for seated practice, stress relief techniques, and supportive prop utilization. Let's explore each day's focus to gain a better understanding

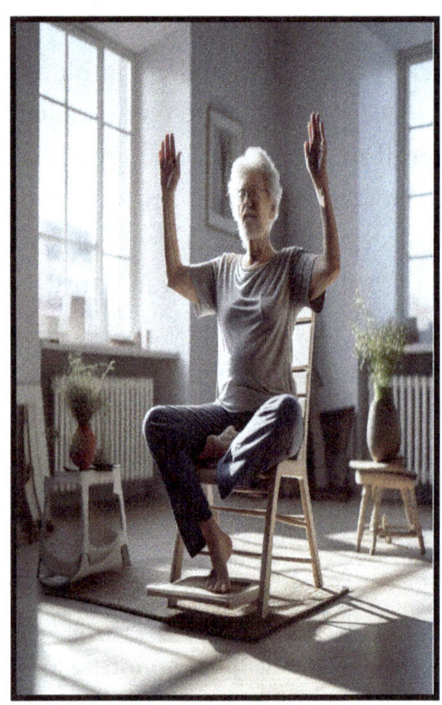

of the suggested approach.

Day 22: Full Body Chair Yoga Flow

On Day 22 of the chair yoga practice plan, you will engage in a full-body chair yoga flow. This sequence aims to promote mobility, flexibility, and strength while focusing on the coordination of breath and movement.

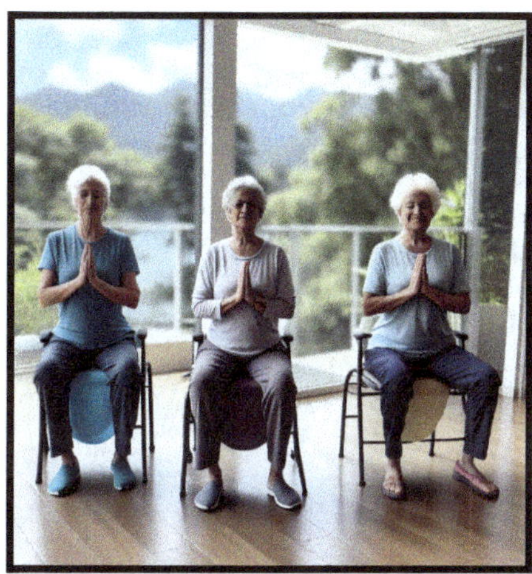

Here's a suggested chair yoga flow that you can incorporate into your practice:

1. **Seated Mountain Pose:**
     - Sit tall in your chair with your feet grounded and your spine elongated.
     - Bring your palms together at heart center, taking a moment to center and ground yourself.
     - On an inhale, extend your arms overhead, lengthening through your torso while maintaining a stable base in the chair.
   - Exhale and bring your hands back to heart center.

2. **Seated Cat-Cow Stretch**:
   - Place your hands on your knees.
   - As you inhale, arch your back and lift your chest (Cow Pose).
   - As you exhale, round your spine, tucking your chin to your chest (Cat Pose).

- Repeat this gentle movement, synchronizing breath with the spinal movements.

3. **Seated Forward Fold**:
   - Sit on the edge of your chair with your feet grounded.
   - On an exhale, hinge at your hips and fold forward, allowing your hands to reach towards your feet or the floor.
   - Feel a gentle stretch along your back and hamstrings. Hold for a few breaths, then slowly return to a seated position as you inhale.

4. **Seated Twist**:
   - Sit tall and place your right hand on the outside of your left knee or thigh.
   - As you inhale, lengthen your spine, and as you exhale, gently twist to the left, using your hand on the knee to deepen the twist.
   - Hold the twist for a few breaths, then return to center and repeat on the other side.

5. **Seated Warrior I:**
   - Extend your right leg forward and bend your left knee, keeping your left foot grounded.
   - Lift your arms overhead, creating a gentle backbend and engaging your core as you lift your chest.

- Hold for a few breaths, then switch to the other side, extending your left leg forward and bending your right knee.

6. **Seated Leg Lifts:**
- Sit towards the front edge of the chair, with your hands gripping the sides for stability.
- Lift one leg at a time, extending it forward and engaging your core.
- Lower the leg back down and repeat with the other leg. This movement helps engage the abdominal muscles and promotes leg strength.

7. **Seated Relaxation**:
- Spend a few moments sitting tall, focusing on your breath and allowing your body to relax.
- Close your eyes if comfortable and bring your attention to the present moment, letting go of any tension or stress.

Throughout this flow, remember to maintain a steady and rhythmic breath, syncing your breath with each movement. This full-body chair yoga flow aims to invigorate your body, promote flexibility, and cultivate a mindful connection between breath and movement while adapting traditional yoga poses to a seated practice. As you move through the sequence, listen to your body and modify the poses as needed to ensure comfort and safety.

Enjoy the holistic benefits of this full-body chair yoga flow on Day 22 of your practice plan.

Day 23: *Seated Sun Salutation*

For Day 23 of the chair yoga practice plan, you will explore a modified version of the traditional Sun Salutation sequence specifically designed for a seated

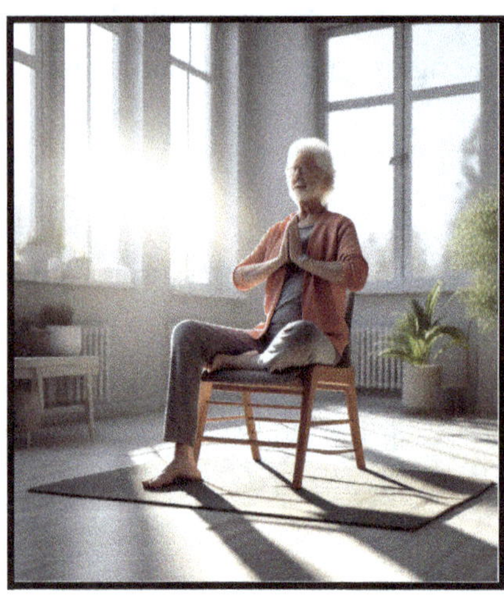

practice. The Seated Sun Salutation aims to invigorate the body, foster flexibility, and synchronize movement with breath, all within the comfort of a chair. Follow the steps below to engage in the Seated Sun Salutation:

1. Seated Mountain Pose:

- Sit tall in your chair, grounding your feet and lengthening your spine.

- Bring your palms together at heart center, taking a moment to center yourself and establish a steady breath.

2. Seated Raised Arms Pose:

- On an inhale, extend your arms overhead, lifting them skyward while maintaining a stable and grounded base in the chair.

- Feel the stretch along your sides and abdomen as you lengthen through your torso.

3. Seated Forward Fold:

- As you exhale, hinge at your hips and fold forward, bringing your hands toward your feet or the floor. Allow your head to relax and feel a gentle stretch along your back and hamstrings.

- Inhale as you slowly rise back to a seated position, lengthening your spine.

4. Seated Half Forward Fold:

- Extend your spine forward, placing your hands on your shins or the sides of your chair.

- Feel a gentle stretch along your spine and the back of your legs; hold for a few breaths before returning to a seated position.

5. Seated Raised Arms Pose:

- Once again, on an inhale, extend your arms overhead, lifting them with a sense of lightness and expansiveness.

6. Seated Mountain Pose:

- Return to your starting position with your palms together at heart center, sitting tall and grounded.

Repeat this sequence, synchronizing each movement with your breath. Each round flows seamlessly into the next, offering a gentle and accessible way to experience the essence of the traditional Sun Salutation while seated. Embrace the rhythm of your breath and movement, cultivating a sense of fluidity and mindfulness throughout the practice.

This modified Seated Sun Salutation sequence serves to energize your body, promote a sense of vitality, and honor the spirit of the traditional Sun Salutation within the context of chair yoga. As always, honor your body's unique needs and comfort levels, modifying the movements as necessary to ensure a safe and enjoyable practice experience.

Engage in the Seated Sun Salutation with a sense of presence and intention, savoring the opportunity to celebrate movement and breath in a seated yoga practice. It's a beautiful way to infuse your day with a touch of yoga's timeless vitality and grace.

Day 24: Chair Yoga Fusion - Mixed Poses

For Day 24 of the chair yoga practice plan, you are invited to explore a fusion of mixed poses tailored to a seated practice. This sequence incorporates a variety of chair yoga postures to promote mobility, flexibility, and mindful movement. Embrace the opportunity to engage in a diverse range of poses while seated in a chair, fostering a sense of well-being and vitality. Follow the sequence below to experience a fusion of mixed chair yoga poses:

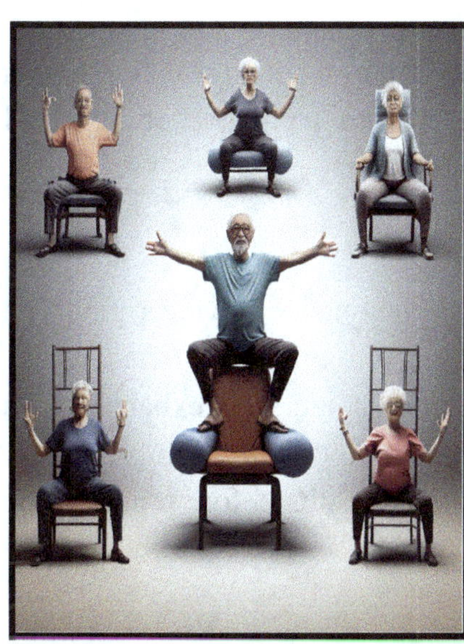

1. **Seated Mountain Pose**:
    - Sit tall in your chair, grounding your feet and lengthening your spine.
    - Bring your palms together at heart center, finding a moment of centered stillness before beginning your sequence.

2. Seated Cat-Cow Stretch:

- On an inhale, arch your back and lift your chest, gazing slightly upward (Cow Pose).

- Exhale and round your spine, tucking your chin toward your chest (Cat Pose).

- Repeat this gentle flowing movement, syncing breath with motion as you explore spinal mobility and flexibility from a seated position.

3. Seated Twist:

- Plant your left hand on the outside of your right thigh while bringing your right hand to the back of the chair.

- Inhale to lengthen your spine, and exhale as you gently twist to the right, gazing over your right shoulder.

- Hold the twist for a few breaths before repeating on the opposite side.

4. Seated Forward Fold:

- Hinge at your hips and fold forward, reaching your hands toward your feet or the floor.

- Embrace a gentle stretch along your back and hamstrings, allowing your head to release and your spine to lengthen.

5. Seated Shoulder Opener:

- Interlace your fingers behind your back, gently opening through the chest and shoulders as you lift your hands away from your body.

- Take a few breaths to explore the sensation of expansion and release in the upper body.

6. **Seated Leg Extension with Forward Fold**:

- Extend one leg forward, flexing your foot, and fold gently over your extended leg.

- Feel a soothing stretch along the back of your extended leg as you breathe into the posture.

- Switch sides and repeat the movement with the opposite leg.

7. **Seated Gentle Twist with Side Bend:**

- Sit tall and place your right hand on the outside of your left knee while reaching your left arm overhead.

- Inhale to lengthen your spine, and exhale as you gently twist to the left while leaning to the right, feeling a side stretch along your left waist.

- Return to center and repeat on the other side.

8. **Seated Meditation with Breath Awareness:**

- Close your eyes and bring your attention to the natural flow of your breath, allowing it to be your focal point for a few moments of seated meditation.

- Embrace a sense of calm and inner stillness as you conclude your fusion of mixed chair yoga poses.

This fusion of mixed chair yoga poses offers a comprehensive exploration of movement and mindful embodiment, catering to the needs of a seated yoga practice. Embrace the opportunity to engage in diverse postures that promote flexibility, mobility, and a sense of well-being while honoring the unique capabilities of your body.

Take time to savor the nourishing effects of each pose and the collective harmony of the sequence as a whole. This fusion serves as a testament to the adaptability and inclusivity of chair yoga, offering a rich and transformative practice experience within a seated framework.

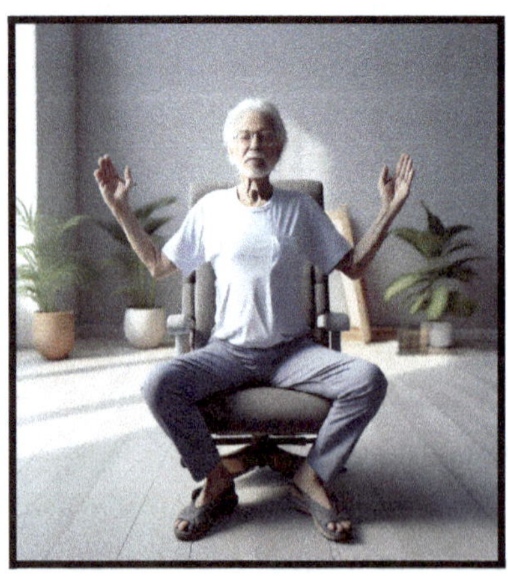

Day 25: Chair Yoga for Stress Relief

For Day 25 of the chair yoga practice plan, you are encouraged to dedicate time to a soothing and rejuvenating session specifically designed for stress relief. This chair yoga sequence aims to promote relaxation, release tension, and cultivate a sense of inner calm through gentle movements and mindful breathing. Embrace the opportunity to nurture your well-being as you engage in the following chair yoga practice for stress relief:

1. **Seated Centering and Breath Awareness**:
   - Sit comfortably in your chair with your feet grounded and your spine tall.
   - Close your eyes and bring your attention to your breath, allowing it to slow and deepen.
   - Spend a few moments centering yourself, focusing on the soothing rhythm of your breath as it flows in and out of your body.

2. **Seated Shoulder Rolls and Neck Stretches**:
   - Gently roll your shoulders up, back, and down, releasing any tension held in the upper body.
   - Perform gentle neck stretches, tilting your head from side to side and forward and backward, moving mindfully and with awareness of any areas of tightness.

3. **Seated Cat-Cow Stretch**:
   - On an inhale, arch your back and lift your chest, gazing slightly upward (Cow Pose).
   - Exhale and round your spine, tucking your chin toward your chest (Cat Pose).

- Repeat this gentle flowing movement, allowing the breath to guide your transitions and inviting a sense of ease into your body.

4. Seated Heart Opener:
- Interlace your fingers behind your lower back, opening through the chest and gently lifting your clasped hands away from your body.
- Take a few deep breaths, feeling a sense of expansion and release in the front of your body.

5. Seated Gentle Twist with Side Bend:
- Place your right hand on the outside of your left knee and your left hand on the armrest or back of the chair.
- Inhale to lengthen your spine, and exhale as you gently twist to the left, feeling a nurturing stretch in your torso.
- Return to center and then lean to the right, feeling a gentle side bend along your left waist.
- Switch sides and repeat the sequence, honoring the gentle release and soothing effect of these movements.

6. Seated Forward Fold:
- Hinge at the hips and fold forward, allowing your hands to rest on your shins, ankles, or the floor.
- Focus on releasing tension in your back and shoulders, breathing deeply as you softy surrender into the posture.

7. Seated Pawanmuktasana (Knee-to-Chest) Variation:

- Hug one knee into your chest, gently rocking from side to side to massage the lower back and promote a sense of comfort and ease.

- Release and repeat the movement with the opposite knee, embracing the nurturing sensation of this gentle self-embrace.

8. Seated Meditation and Deep Breathing:

- Close your eyes and practice deep diaphragmatic breathing, allowing each breath to be full and nourishing.

- Embrace a few moments of seated meditation, directing your attention inward and nurturing a sense of inner peace and tranquility.

Conclude your chair yoga practice for stress relief with a few moments of stillness, acknowledging the restorative effects of your session. Embrace the opportunity to reset and replenish your energy, allowing the soothing movements and mindful breathwork to create a sense of inner balance and calm.

This chair yoga sequence for stress relief serves as a nurturing and supportive practice, offering an accessible avenue to release tension and promote emotional well-being. By engaging in these gentle movements and mindful breathwork, you honor your holistic well-being and cultivate resilience in the face of stress. Embrace the restorative power of chair yoga as you prioritize your relaxation and inner harmony.

Day 26: Chair Yoga for Better Sleep

For Day 26 of the chair yoga practice plan, it's time to focus on a calming and restorative chair yoga session

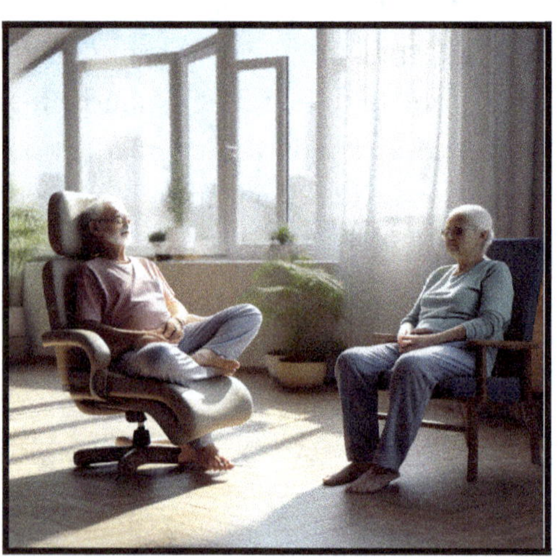

designed to promote better sleep. The gentle movements and mindful breathing techniques incorporated into this sequence aim to relax the body and mind, ease muscle tension, and create an environment conducive to restful sleep. Embrace the opportunity to nurture your well-being as you engage in the following chair yoga practice for better sleep:

1. **Seated Centering and Breath Awareness**:

- Find a comfortable seated position in your chair, grounding your feet and elongating your spine.

- Close your eyes and take a few moments to center yourself, bringing awareness to your breath and allowing its rhythm to slow and deepen.

2. **Seated Neck and Shoulder Release**:

- Gently roll your shoulders and perform neck stretches, releasing any tension held in these areas to promote relaxation.

3. **Seated Side Stretch and Gentle Twists**:

- Inhale to lengthen your spine, and as you exhale, gently lean to one side, feeling a soothing stretch along the opposite side of your torso.

- Return to center and then perform a gentle twist, encouraging a sense of release and openness in your spine and back.

4. **Seated Forward Fold and Half Sun Salutation**:

- Hinge forward from your hips and fold gently, allowing your hands to rest on your legs or the floor, focusing on releasing tension and calming the mind.

- Perform a modified half Sun Salutation, flowing through gentle movements to encourage relaxation and ease in your body.

5. Seated Figure Four Stretch:

- Cross one ankle over the opposite knee, gently pressing down on the raised knee to feel a soothing stretch in your hip and glute muscles.

- Switch sides and repeat the stretch, honoring the nurturing sensation of this release.

6. Seated Cat-Cow Stretch and Pawanmuktasana (Knee-to-Chest) Variation:

- Flow through gentle seated Cat-Cow movements, allowing your breath to guide the transition as you nurture your spine and promote relaxation.

- Hug one knee into your chest, gently rocking from side to side to massage the lower back and prepare the body for restful sleep.

7. Seated Meditation and Deep Breathing:

- Close your eyes and practice deep, diaphragmatic breathing, allowing each breath to be a source of calm and comfort.

- Embrace a few moments of seated meditation, directing your attention inward and nurturing a sense of inner tranquility.

8. Progressive Muscle Relaxation:

- Starting from your toes, consciously tense and then relax each muscle group as you work your way up through your body, promoting a sense of physical and mental release.

Conclude your chair yoga practice for better sleep with a few moments of stillness, acknowledging the calming and centering effects of your session. Embrace the opportunity to create a peaceful space for rest and rejuvenation, allowing the soothing movements and mindfulness practices to prepare you for a restorative night's sleep.

This chair yoga sequence for better sleep offers a gentle and supportive practice, providing an accessible avenue to unwind and nurture your sleep quality. By engaging in these calming movements and incorporating mindful breathwork, you honor your holistic well-being and cultivate the conditions for restful sleep. Embrace the restorative power of chair yoga as you prioritize your relaxation and prepare your body and mind for a night of deep, rejuvenating sleep.

Day 27: Incorporating Props for Support

On Day 27 of the chair yoga practice plan, we will incorporate props to enhance support and comfort during your practice. Props can play a crucial role in making yoga more accessible, providing stability, promoting proper alignment, and accommodating individual needs. In this session, we will utilize props to facilitate a mindful and nurturing chair yoga practice. Here's a chair yoga sequence that integrates props for added support:

1. **Seated Centering and Breath Awareness**:
   - Begin in a comfortable seated position, grounding your feet and elongating your spine. You may consider using a cushion or folded blanket for additional support and comfort.

2. **Supported Seated Mountain Pose:**
   - Place a yoga block or a folded blanket between your thighs to encourage engagement of the inner thighs and support proper alignment. As you sit tall, bring your palms together at heart center and gently extend your arms overhead, feeling the support and stability provided by the prop.

3. **Gentle Shoulder Opener with Strap or Scarf**:
   - Hold a yoga strap or a scarf with both hands, allowing your arms to gently extend behind your back. This supported shoulder opener can help release tension and promote openness in the chest and shoulders.

4. **Seated Twists with Prop Support:**

- Hold the back of your chair with one hand and gently twist, using the chair as a support for your twist. This can enhance the depth of the twist while providing stability.

5. Gentle Seated Forward Fold with Prop Support:

- Rest your forearms on a bolster, cushion, or stack of folded blankets on your lap as you fold forward from your hips. This gentle supported forward fold can promote relaxation and release tension in the back and hips.

6. Supported Seated Pawanmuktasana (Knee-to-Chest) Pose:

- Hug your knees to your chest, utilizing a bolster or cushion to support your thighs. This variation provides a nurturing stretch for the lower back and can create a sense of comfort and ease.

7. Reclined Leg Extension with Prop Support:

- If accessible, extend your legs and support the backs of your thighs with a bolster or folded blanket. This gentle supported leg extension can promote relaxation and help release tension in the legs and lower back.

8. Supported Seated Meditation and Breathwork:

- Sit comfortably on your chair, utilizing props such as cushions or bolsters to support your seated position.

Close your eyes, focus on deep, diaphragmatic breathing, and embrace a few moments of seated meditation for relaxation and centering.

9. **Closing Relaxation**:

- Conclude your practice by reclining back in your chair, utilizing any additional props for comfort and support. Allow your body to rest and relax, savoring the nurturing effects of your chair yoga session.

By integrating props into your chair yoga practice, you provide yourself with the necessary support to enhance comfort, stability, and alignment. Embracing the use of props fosters an inclusive and adaptable yoga practice, ensuring that individuals with diverse needs and abilities can experience the nurturing benefits of yoga. By utilizing props mindfully, you honor your body's unique requirements and create a supportive environment for your chair yoga practice.

Incorporating props into chair yoga promotes accessibility and encourages practitioners to tailor their practice to suit their individual needs, ensuring that yoga remains an inclusive and welcoming practice for all. Embrace the supportive nature of props as you cultivate a mindful and nurturing chair yoga practice tailored to your comfort and well-being.

Day 28: Celebration and Reflection

On Day 28 of your chair yoga practice plan, we will focus on celebration and reflection. This session is

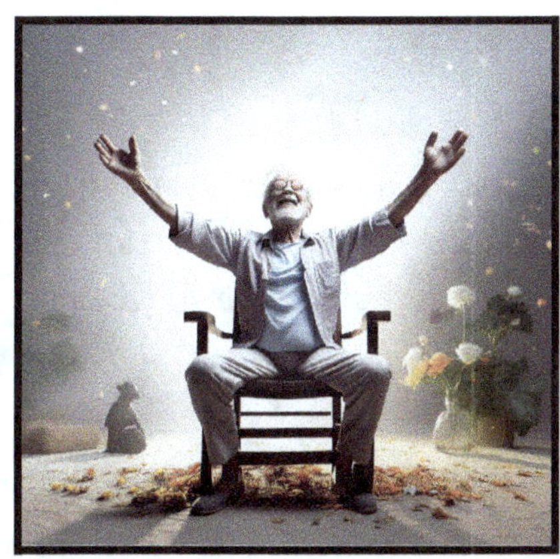

designed to provide an opportunity for you to honor your journey, celebrate your achievements, and reflect on the benefits and growth you've experienced throughout your chair yoga practice. It's essential to acknowledge the progress you've made and the positive effects that consistent practice has had on your well-being. Here's a suggested framework for your celebration and reflection chair yoga session:

1. **Setting the Space**:
   - Create a calming and inviting environment for your practice by dimming the lights, playing soft, soothing music, and perhaps lighting a candle to foster a reflective atmosphere.

2. **Gratitude Meditation**:

- Begin your session with a gratitude meditation, expressing thanks for the ability to engage in chair yoga, the support you've received, and the positive impact it has had on your life. Take a few moments to cultivate a sense of gratitude in your heart.

3. Gentle Movement and Breathwork:

- Engage in gentle seated movements and deep, mindful breathing to cultivate a sense of calm and mindfulness. Allow the breath to guide your movements and help center your focus.

4. Reflection and Journaling:

- Take some time for quiet reflection and journaling. Consider the following prompts:

- How has chair yoga positively impacted your physical well-being?

- In what ways has chair yoga supported your emotional and mental health?

- What achievements or progress have you noticed throughout your chair yoga journey?

- Are there any insights or revelations you've gained from your practice?

- How has chair yoga enhanced your overall quality of life?

- Take the opportunity to write down your thoughts and reflections, capturing the significance of your chair yoga experience.

5. Celebration through Movement:

- Engage in celebratory movements such as gentle seated dancing or flowing with joyful and expressive arm movements. Allow yourself to embody a sense of celebration and joy through movement.

6. Seated Heart-Opening Poses:

- Practice seated heart-opening poses such as Supported Seated Mountain Pose, extending the arms overhead with an open heart to symbolize embracing the positive energy and growth from your chair yoga practice.

7. Loving-Kindness Meditation:

- Conclude your practice with a loving-kindness meditation, directing well-wishes and compassion towards yourself, your loved ones, and all beings. Embrace the spirit of kindness and positivity as you close your session.

8. Closing Reflection:

- Sit quietly for a few moments, allowing the feelings of celebration and reflection to settle within you. Acknowledge the significance of this practice and the positive impact it has had on your well-being.

9. Affirmations and Positive Intentions:

Conclude your celebration and reflection by setting affirmations or positive intentions for the days ahead. Embrace empowering thoughts and aspirations as you transition from your practice back into your daily life.

This Day 28 session is an opportunity to honor the journey you've undertaken and recognize the transformative effects of your chair yoga practice. Embracing celebration and reflection allows you to fully appreciate the positive changes and growth that have emerged from your commitment to chair yoga. By acknowledging your progress and expressing gratitude for the benefits you've experienced, you reinforce the value of your practice and cultivate a sense of fulfillment and contentment.

Chair yoga has the power to foster physical, emotional, and mental well-being, and through celebration and reflection, you affirm the positive impact it has on your life. This practice is an expression of self-care and self-compassion, ensuring that you honor the dedication and effort you've invested in your well-being through chair yoga. Celebrate the journey, reflect on the growth, and carry the positive energy and insights gained from this practice into the days ahead.

Conclusion:

I want to express my deepest appreciation for your commitment to your chair yoga practice and for embracing the practices outlined in this plan. Your dedication and enthusiasm reflect a genuine investment in your overall well-being. I also want to acknowledge the support and encouragement you've received from those around you, and extend gratitude to the individuals and resources that have contributed to your learning and growth during this chair yoga practice plan.

As you move forward on your journey, may you continue to embrace the transformative power of chair yoga, fostering holistic well-being and vitality. Your dedication to enhancing your health and wellness through chair yoga is truly commendable, and I encourage you to carry the positive energy, insights, and benefits gained from this practice into your daily life.

Lastly, I want to express my sincere gratitude to you for choosing this chair yoga practice plan as a resource for your well-being journey. If you've found value in this plan, I kindly ask that you consider leaving a review. Your feedback can provide valuable insights for others and also inspire fellow practitioners to explore the transformative benefits of chair yoga.

Your support and feedback are immensely appreciated and can help others discover the positive impact that chair yoga can have on their lives. Your review has the potential to uplift and guide others on their wellness journey, and I am grateful for your consideration.

Thank you for choosing this chair yoga practice plan, and I'm truly honored to have been a part of your wellness experience. Wishing you continued fulfillment, balance, and wellness on your chair yoga journey and beyond. Thank you for your trust, and may your journey be filled with positivity, growth, and well-being.